Spinal
Manipulation
Made Simple

Spinal Manipulation Made Simple

A Manual of Soft Tissue Techniques

Jeffrey Maitland

Photographs by Kelley Kirkpatrick

North Atlantic Books
Berkeley, California

Spinal Manipulation Made Simple

Published by
North Atlantic Books
P.O. Box 12327
Berkeley, California 94712

Cover photograph by Brandy Wilkins
Cover and book design by Paula Morrison
Printed in the United States of America

Spinal Manipulation Made Simple is sponsored by the Society for the Study of Native Arts and Sciences, a nonprofit educational corporation whose goals are to develop an educational and crosscultural perspective linking various scientific, social, and artistic fields; to nurture a holistic view of arts, sciences, humanities, and healing; and to publish and distribute literature on the relationship of mind, body, and nature.

Library of Congress Cataloging-in-Publication Data

Maitland, Jeffrey, 1943–
    Spinal manipulation made simple : a manual of soft tissue techniques / by Jeffrey Maitland.
        p. cm.
    ISBN 1-55643-352-2 (trade paper : alk. paper)
    1. Spinal adjustment—Handbooks, manuals, etc. 2. Manipulation (Therapeutics)—Handbooks, manuals, etc. I. Title.

RZ265.S64 M35 2000
615.8'2—dc21

                                                                00-041133

        4 5 6 7 8 9 DATA 08 07 06 05 04

ACKNOWLEDGMENTS

Spinal Manipulation Made Simple answers a question that many somatic manual therapists have pondered: Is it possible to release spinal fixations without resorting to high-velocity, low-amplitude thrusting techniques employed by osteopaths and chiropractors? This book delineates my very straightforward and simple technical solution to this problem. But simple solutions often have complex histories that result from the confluence of many disparate influences. There are so many people that have helped me find my way that I would be disrespectful and remiss if I didn't try to thank some of them.

With respect to somatic therapy, the most important influence on the evolution of my approach comes from the many people at the Rolf Institute who labored in the service of teaching me the theory and art of the Rolfing®[1] method of Structural Integration and how to teach it. I am especially indebted to the teaching and gifts of senior teachers Jan Sultan and Michael Salveson and I want to acknowledge their untiring dedication to the education of Rolfers. Their influence can be found in various places throughout this book. I am also very grateful for what I learned from Emmett Hutchins and Peter Melchior when they were still members of the Rolf Institute. My understanding of the functional side of somatic therapy has benefitted greatly from the work of the movement teachers at the Rolf Institute, especially from the following people: Hubert Godard, Jane Harrington, Megan James, Vivian Jaye, Gael Ohlgren, and Heather Wing. I also want to acknowledge John Cottingham, physical therapist, researcher, and Rolfer not only for his support, generosity of heart, and sparkling intellect, but also for his sensational research on holistic manual and movement therapy. I feel privileged to have worked with him and to have been able to publish two articles with him. His research is not only elegant, but some of the best on holistic manual therapy.

I have greatly benefitted, both professionally and personally, from the wonderful work of osteopathy. I owe a special debt of gratitude to the guidance and generosity of my friend and mentor, the late Dr. Walter Wirth, D.O. His brilliant work and teaching changed not only my body, but the direction of my work as a somatic practitioner. I am also grateful for the introduction to the mysteries of the cranium and indirect touch that I received from Dr. John Upledger, D.O. early in my development as a Rolfer. I feel especially fortunate to have been able to train with the Upledger Institute and Didier Prat, D.O. in the revolutionary Visceral Manipulation developed by Jean-Pierre Barral, D.O. Many thanks to Dr. Marilyn Wells, D.O. and the other Arizona osteopaths with whom I have had the great pleasure to associate. I have learned more than I can say from a great number of books on osteopathy, but I particularly appreciate the work of Phillip Greenman, D.O.

I also want to thank Dr. Joseph DeBriun, D.C. and Dr. L. Jon Porman, D.C. for their excellent work on my joints and for introducing me to the principles and practice of Dynamic Chiropractic. Although I do not employ chiropractic technique in my practice, I have found their approach to motion testing and understanding spinal fixation invaluable.

I am by instinct and training a philosopher above all else. Philosophy has many faces, but the one I am most attracted to concerns the nature of being. Another important aspect of philosophy consists in exposing and examining the veracity of the presuppositions that inform our every attempt to understand the nature of reality. This aspect has led some thinkers to dub philosophy "the queen of the sciences." Although it may not be immediately obvious, these two concerns are at work in the background of this manual. To all the philosophers who have contributed so much to my growth over the years I give heartfelt thanks.

One of the greatest practical philosophers with whom I have had the good fortune to study is my Zen teacher. I caught my first glimpse of how the body speaks to an open heart while cuddling my infant daughters. But this truth about the activity of being did not really blossom until it was simultaneously articulated and manifested by my Roshi. His influence continues to alter the course of my life and work. Even the Oxford English Dictionary cannot supply enough words to express the depth of my gratitude to him. I remember asking him, "How do you heal people?" With a spacious imperturbability that showed no hesitation, he said, "Ahh, you must become one with them!" His simple answer portends a great depth. Today, twenty years later, I think I am just beginning to grasp the wisdom he demonstrated. I hope some small part of his profound teachings has also found its way into this book.

I want to thank Kelley Kirkpatrick for her wonderful photographs that so clearly demonstrate my techniques. Her skill, patience, and aesthetic sensitivity are a gift. Also many thanks go to David Robinson, Rolfer, who generously agreed to be the model.

Finally, I want to give thanks to my pain for leading me to a new and better life. But most of all, I want to give my deepest bow of gratitude to my detractors. From them I have learned the impossible.

Note

1. Rolfing® is a service mark of the Rolf Institute of Structural Integration.

ILLUSTRATIONS

Permission to use their illustrations was granted from the following publications:

The illustrations of the spine in forward and backward bending and the dysfunctional vertebrae (Figures 2.1, 2.2, and 2.3) come from Greenman, Phillip E. *The Principles of Manual Medicine*, second edition. Baltimore, Maryland: Williams and Wilkins, 1996, figures 5.24 and 5.25 on p. 61 and figure 6.1 on p. 67.

The illustration of rib tender points (Figure 9.5) comes from DiGiovanna, Eileen L. and Schiowitz, Stanley. *An Osteopathic Approach to Diagnosis and Treatment*. New York, New York: Williams and Wilkins, 1991, figures 17.7 and 17.10 on pp. 261-262.

The following illustrations come from Kapandji, I. A *The Physiology of the Joints*, Vol Three. New York, New York: Churchill Livingstone, 1974.

> Figure 4.2 is 34 on p. 193.
> Figure 7.14 and 10.11 are 8, 9, and 10 on p. 61.
> Figure 7.13 is 2 on p. 11.
> Figure 8.1 is 11 and 12 on p.63.
> Figure10.3 is 11 and 12 on p. 63.
> Figure 10.7 is 75 p.233.
> Figure 10.10 is 6 on p. 59 and 8, 9, 10 on p. 61.

The photograph in Figure 8.3 displaying an posteriorly tilted and anteriorly shifted pelvis comes from Kendall, Florence Peterson and McCreary, Elizabeth Kendall. *Muscles: Testing and Function*, Third edition. Baltimore, Maryland: Williams and Wilkins, 1983, p. 284.

The illustration of the of the Ideal Body (Figure 10.8) comes from Kendall, Florence Peterson and McCreary, Elizabeth Kendall. *Muscles: Testing and Function*, Third edition. Baltimore: (Williams and Wilkins), 1983, p. 280.

The illustration of the rib/vertebral complex (Figure 9.1) comes from Schultz, R. Louis and Feitis, Rosemary. *The Endless Web*. Berkeley, California: North Atlantic Books, 1996, figure 9.1 is 8.5 on p. 30.

The illustration of the possible positions of the sciatic nerve in relation to the piriformis muscle (Figure 10.4) comes from Ward, Robert, ed. *Foundations for Osteopathic Medicine*. Baltimore, Maryland: Williams and Wilkins, 1997, figure 10.4 is 49.6 p. 606.

The illustration of the ideal spine (Figure 10.9) comes from Rolf, Ida P. *Rolfing: The Integration of Human Structures*. Santa Monica: Dennis-Landman Publishers, 1977, figure 10.9 is 13.3 on p. 209.

CONTENTS

INTRODUCTION

THIS BOOK GREW OUT OF MY BACK PAIN AND MY DEEP APPRECIATION FOR the somatic manual therapists who allowed me to heal and find a new life. I remember all too well the day my back "went out" for the first time. I was 27 years old, fresh out of graduate school, and into my second semester of teaching philosophy at Purdue University. Feeling the need to get into better shape, I had begun a rather thoughtless program of exercise. A few days later, I awoke to a nasty pain in my lower back confined to an area about the size of a 50-cent piece. By noon I couldn't stand up straight. I was pitched forward at a 45-degree angle and forced to lean on a broom handle to move about. My wife arrived home from running errands to find me in this deplorable condition. She drove me to the local emergency room where I was prodded and poked, and then sent home with muscle relaxants. The muscle relaxants were useless; their only effect was to turn me into a stuporous version of the local village idiot. When the effects wore off, I immediately flushed my medications down the toilet. That day marked the beginning of a seven-year search for relief.

At first I tried the conventional medical approach. On the first visit to my doctor, an orthopedic surgeon, I was informed I had back pain because human beings were not designed to stand upright. "What a bizarre theory!" I thought. "Does he think that I would not have developed back pain if I had spent my life crawling around on my hands and knees? Obviously we are not designed for that way of getting about either." I knew better than to express my objections to his theory because he, like too many other authoritarian practitioners, made up specious explanations at the drop of a hat. Besides, I was in pain, and at that moment in my life he was my only hope. I certainly didn't want him angry with me. He then sent me to a physical therapist who gave me a set of useless exercises. Over time

my pain subsided and I began jogging in the naive belief that I was helping my back problem.

Over the next few years my back regularly "went out." When the pain
was at its worst, I made another appointment with my doctor. Even though
I had no pain radiating down either leg, he informed me, without the
benefit of X-rays or any other kind of images of my back, that I had a
bulging disk, and said, "You know, if I have to see you too often, we are
going to have to do surgery." His ultimatum was compelling and I drew
the only conclusion I could—I would never go to see him again.

"Surely," I thought, "somebody must understand how backs work, why
they get in trouble, and how they can be helped." A friend recommended
that I go to a chiropractor who had helped her. I made an appointment.
His secretary applied ultrasound to my low back and then he "adjusted"
it. He sold me a back brace and after a few weeks of his treatment, my pain
began to subside. I would make an appointment every time my back flared
up. Unfortunately, even though my chiropractor could ease my pain, he
could never keep me that way. After many treatments my neck also began
to cause me trouble and every session I had to remind him to "adjust" my
neck. I continued to jog and my pain continued to get worse.

A number of years later I allowed another chiropractor to strap me
onto a table that looked like it had been built in the last century. As he
tightened the straps I felt vaguely uneasy and had a momentary vision of
myself as a victim of the Crusades. As he slowly turned the crank, I was
tortuously and painfully stretched. I could barely stand afterwards and I
soon developed a horrible case of sciatica. If you have never experienced
this pain, you never want to. It is like having the world's worst toothache
in your butt and legs. So I knew I had to find another way.

While I was on sabbatical from Purdue, on the recommendation of
friends I made an appointment with a very talented Rolfer. To make a
long process short, after thirty five or so sessions with a number of other
Rolfers and with the additional help of a gifted osteopath, I was finally
freed of my back pain. I subsequently became a Rolfer and then a Rolfing teacher.

As my understanding and ability as a Rolfer grew, my frustration with
certain aspects of the traditional approach to Rolfing also grew. Old style
Rolfing was often too painful and much too general to properly handle

local areas of immobility and pain. Before becoming a Rolfer, I had been practicing Zen meditation intensely for a number of years and had somewhat unintentionally developed the ability to feel energy in and around my clients' bodies. Unfortunately the heavy pressure I was taught to use when applying the techniques of Rolfing made it impossible for me to feel the subtle energy connections throughout the body. For a number of years I experimented with trying to find a gentler approach that would not sacrifice the profound structural changes for which Rolfing is known. I bumbled along until I finally learned how to feel the energies of the body while still applying the heavy pressure often required by Rolfing. My confidence grew as I realized that I was able to apply a full range of pressures, from very light to very heavy, without causing unnecessary discomfort to the client or sacrificing the goals of Rolfing. These explorations also allowed me to penetrate more deeply into and through the body's tangled webs of fascial and energetic confusion.

My clients were happy because I was getting better results without causing unnecessary discomfort. Many reported that their experience of massage was actually more uncomfortable than the way I Rolfed. I was feeling better about my work because I was also able to be very specific without losing sight of the whole. Unfortunately, I did not remain content for long. As if some universal principle were being worked out in my life that nobody had informed me about, the better a Rolfer I became, the more difficult my client's problems became.

While I was training to become a teacher of advanced Rolfing I learned that two senior teachers, Jan Sultan and Michael Salveson, were already in the process of trying to solve many of the same problems that I had been struggling with. I was able to build on their insights and my investigations revealed that many of the traditional Rolfing techniques were all too often incapable of releasing facet restrictions in the spine and other joints of the body. As Rolfing instructors, we had no interest in teaching the high-velocity, low-amplitude thrusting techniques pioneered by osteopaths and later adopted by chiropractors. Since Rolfing is a form of myofascial manipulation and education, we wanted our techniques to look and feel like a variation of our already established approach to soft-tissue manipulation. Crudely stated, high-velocity techniques are designed to "pop" joint fixations free, but they look and feel nothing like Rolfing.

We had explored other soft-tissue techniques similar to ours, but soon realized that they were incapable of producing the global structural changes of Rolfing. We also discovered that many of the popularized myofascial-release techniques that were misappropriated from osteopathy and Rolfing tended to merely "unwind" the tissue around the joint without ever releasing the actual fixation. Our goal was to find methods of mobilizing joint fixations that were consistent with the way Rolfing works with soft tissue, but we had no interest in importing techniques from other disciplines. After studying how joints work and become restricted, I experimented with and finally managed to develop a range of soft-tissue techniques that effectively release joint fixation without resorting to high-velocity thrusting techniques or any other techniques developed in other systems of manual therapy. These soft-tissue techniques, coupled with an understanding of how the spine gets in and out of trouble comprise the content of this book.

Like so many other people struggling to overcome debilitating back pain, I was worked on by many different practitioners from many different schools of therapy. I noticed that a few were astonishingly more effective than others and that they all had similar qualities and abilities that were missing in the average therapist. You will often hear the average practitioner boast that his technique or approach is so much better than all the others because he doing something remarkably and uniquely different from everyone else. But my experience as a patient and teacher of manual therapy led me to just the opposite conclusion: what makes for a really good practitioner is not what is different about his or her approach, but what he or she shares in common with all great practitioners in every discipline. In the end there is nothing unique about being unique, because the power is not in what is unique, but in what is common.

These qualities are fairly easy to state, but not so easy to teach. All of the gifted practitioners who worked with me exhibited an uncanny perceptual vitality and sensitivity that allowed them to see and feel the details of my problems with an exquisite specificity and mastery of technique that never lost sight of my whole person. They were capable of releasing local areas of dysfunction in a way that benefitted my entire body. They released my symptoms without ever getting caught in the trap of chasing them and they were always able to track how their local manipulations cascaded throughout my whole body. As a result, they almost always knew where to work next and they rarely drove problems to other areas of my body. Since my body was constantly changing and improving under their care, they rarely repeated the same session. But most importantly, because they could keep the whole of me in view and affect the whole as they addressed local areas of my body, their work often produced far-reaching and long-lasting changes.

All of these practitioners were also well-educated and well-versed in their disciplines. They had a thorough and detailed knowledge that they continually expanded through further study and research. Part of what made them masters of their arts was their daunting knowledge, their commitment to always learning more, and a most remarkable mastery of technique. But there was another, more elusive, factor that contributed to their mastery—their way of being. At least for the duration of each session, they lived their art with a clarity, compassion, and openness quite beyond everyday life. I felt that my being and pain were seen and understood. I was not treated like a specimen with a problem who was in need of some sort of outside intervention that forced me to measure up to some objective standard of normality. Their uncanny perception, exquisite discrimination, and sense of touch were not rooted in any sort of objective, judgmental separation from me, but in a deeply felt participatory understanding free of conflict, grandiosity, and self-importance. They never tried to convince me that they knew what was best for me or that only they had the answer to my problems. If I didn't respond to their treatment as they expected, they didn't make me feel like it was my fault and were always willing to try another approach or refer me to other practitioners. Unlike so many practitioners who only chased symptoms while paying lip service to a holistic approach, they were truly holistic practitioners.

This way of being, not the mere accumulation of techniques, is both the source of all healing and the limitless heart of life itself. Working this way is not a matter of going into an altered state, but of returning to our senses, to our native condition free of the contaminations and conflicts of self and culture. Once we are freed from our conflicts, we see and feel the world differently, and we no longer stand apart from what we sense. We live and perceive our world with a participatory sensorial affinity that gently embraces and is embraced by both soma and nature. There is a wisdom and spacious clarity that arises from resting in our primordial unconflicted state—without it a therapist is but a mere technician; but with it amazing things are possible.

For this wisdom to evolve into a healing ability, however, it must also be coupled with the right kind of rationality and objective knowledge that is then fully integrated into the somatic intelligence of the therapist—knowledge and wisdom must go hand in hand. To paraphrase Kant: wisdom without knowledge is blind and knowledge without wisdom is empty. Since I have already discussed the nature of transformation in my book *Spacious Body*, I will not dwell on this way of being here, I only mention it because it is so immensely important. Every practitioner has probably experienced moments of this spacious openness, in which every intervention produces almost magical and effortless results. It is, after all, the heart of all healing. Through its cultivation the healer heals herself and becomes effortlessly more effective in healing others.

While no less important than articulating the healer's way of being, this book is not so ambitious. It is rather a practical manual of techniques for treating the spine. It offers all manual therapists some of the knowledge and specificity of technique that is required to treat a number of different kinds of somatic dysfunctions that they see every day in their practices.

However, knowledge and specificity of technique, is not the be-all and end-all of therapy. It is one thing to know how to apply techniques and it is quite another to know when and in what order to apply them. Beyond the mere application of technique there are the three fundamental questions of therapy: "What do I do first, What do I do next, and When am I finished?" Answering these questions to the benefit of our clients is crucial for any holistic approach. However, as important as understanding these considerations is to the development of every practitioner, this book is also not a treatise on the clinical decision process, but a manual of techniques.

The mastery of technique is important for many obvious reasons, not the least of which is the benefit it provides for our clients. But there is another benefit for the practitioner who puts the time and effort into learning how to effectively apply technique: this mastery is one of the necessary stepping stones for cultivating the healer's way of being. Just as practicing scales can be preparatory for the inspired performance of music, so too can practicing techniques become part of the cultivation of the healer's way of being.

No matter what form of manual therapy you were trained in, and regardless of whether you work with a corrective or holistic approach, you will find these techniques deceptively simple to apply and yet highly effective in dealing with most forms of back pain. The techniques all arose from my frustration with my inability to resolve the more difficult back problems that I was seeing in my practice. After I created these techniques I tested them in my practice, classes, and in collaboration with my colleagues, Jan Sultan and Michael Salveson, at the Rolf Institute.

Understanding this book requires a working knowledge of the anatomy of the muscular and skeletal systems. I discuss anatomy where it is relevant, but in the simplest of terms. My goal is to give you the skills you need to evaluate and immediately treat your patients. There are many wonderful books available that go into considerable detail regarding manual therapy and I see no need to repeat what has already been said well. The texts I have found most useful are included in the bibliography.

1

Our Fine Spine: The Backbone of Structural Integrity

F YOUR BACK HAS EVER "GONE OUT," THE EASE WITH WHICH YOU GO about your life goes right out the window with it. And you are not alone— at least 80 million Americans are in the same fix. Many make the mistake of thinking that when their pain disappears their problem also goes away. But experienced clinicians know that this belief is based on an illusion. We could term the confusion of the experience of pain with the problem causing the pain the "fallacy of misplaced hope." A facet restriction can exist at a subclinical level, showing no obvious signs of pain, and then suddenly rear its painful countenance at the most inopportune times. You arise from a chair to greet a friend and suddenly there's that stabbing pain in your back again. Back pain can come and go, but the problem almost always remains. And if left untreated, it often gets worse as time and gravity take their unforgiving toll on our bodies.

Whole disciplines and theories of manual therapy have been created based on the idea that the spine is the most important and sometimes the only area of the body that needs to be treated. As naive as that view is, it is certainly not hard to appreciate its appeal. You don't need a lot of research to understand that if you cannot treat spinal dysfunctions, you are incapable of helping many people. If you are a holistic practitioner trying to provide higher and higher levels of organization and balance for your clients and you cannot release people from their spinal dysfunctions, then your grandest notions of what can be achieved for them will not be realized. There is no doubt about it: understanding and success-fully treating the spine is important to every somatic practitioner, no mat-ter what your point of view.

In order to be effective when you attempt to release a painful joint, you need to know how the joint works when it's normal and how it works when it's in trouble—and how to tell the difference. In order to experi-ence what we are going to be discussing before you read a lot of theory, here is a simple exercise you can do with your own spine.

Stand up and place your thumbs on your spine over the transverse processes (TP) of L4 or L5. Don't worry too much at this point about how accurate you are. Just use your thumbs to make your best guess. Now sidebend (or laterally flex) to your left. When you sidebend to the left, the left side of your lumbar spine will be concave and the right will be con-vex (Figure 1.1). Notice what happens under your thumbs. As you sidebend to your left, your right thumb is forced posteriorly a bit while your left thumb sinks anteriorly a little. Now sidebend the other way and notice that just the opposite occurs: your left thumb is pushed a little posteriorly and your right thumb sinks anteriorly.

What you are feeling is your vertebra rotate as you sidebend. The con-vention for describing rotation is to describe the direction in which the anterior face of the vertebra turns. So while standing or sitting, if you sidebend right, your vertebra will rotate left, and if you sidebend left, your vertebra will rotate right. Sidebending is difficult to feel at first and not something you need to be concerned with at this point. But rotation is easy to palpate. As you will soon see, by knowing the direction in which a vertebra is rotated you can gather lots of the necessary information for dealing with a painful back.

If you have a history of back trouble, you may notice that the vertebral movement you are monitoring with your thumbs is not exactly the same as you sidebend from side to side. This discovery may be no surprise to you—it probably means you have a facet restriction that is inhibiting nor-mal motion through the area you are palpating. If one of the facets is restricted, you will feel the vertebra rotate more as you sidebend one way and less as you sidebend the other. If you feel rotation more in one direc-tion than the other and you haven't had a history of back trouble, don't panic. Perhaps you haven't placed fingers in quite the right area or maybe

2

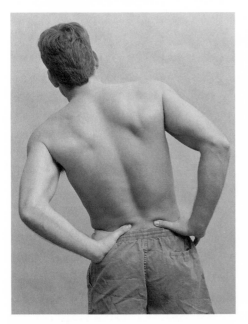 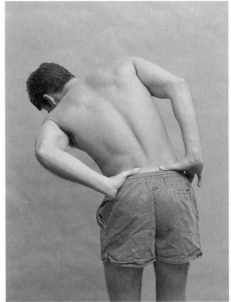

Figure 1.1   *Figure 1.2*

you are having trouble clearly differentiating between what the vertebra is doing and how the soft tissues are responding. In some people the tone of the musculature along the sides of the spine is not the same and as a result each side responds differently to sidebending. Of course, it could mean that you do have some sort of facet restriction that hasn't reached your awareness through the attention-getting medium of pain. But again don't panic, we will learn how to deal with these problems a little later.

What you have learned so far is that sidebending and rotation are always coupled. What you are about to feel next is that they are not always coupled the same way in the thoracic and lumbar spines. Stand up again and place your thumbs on either L4 or L5. If you have a history of back pain and your back is presently in trouble you may not want to try this next exercise. But if you are game, first bend way forward and then sidebend to the left (Figure 1.2). As you sidebend left you will notice that the left transverse process pushes your thumb a little posteriorly and on the right transverse process your other thumb sinks anteriorly a bit. What you are feeling can be described by saying that as you sidebend left in forward bending your vertebra rotates left. Now, while you are still in the forward bent position, sidebend right and you will notice that your vertebra rotates right. Next, straighten up and then back bend. In the back-bent position, sidebend right and left, and notice that your vertebra behaves the same way as it did in the forward bent position: as you sidebend left, your vertebra rotates left and as you sidebend right your vertebra rotates right.

Standing or sitting with the spine comfortably straight is called the neutral position In neutral position the facets do not engage when you sidebend. In the non-neutral positions of forward bending and backward bending the facets of the thoracic and lumbar spines do get engaged and their relationship alters the way the vertebrae rotate. What you have learned through direct palpatory experience are two important facts about the thoracic and lumbar spines: 1) in neutral position, sidebending and rotation are always oppositely coupled and 2) in the non-neutral positions of forward and backward bending, sidebending and rotation are always coupled to the same side. So in neutral position when you right sidebend, your vertebra rotates left and when you left sidebend, your vertebra rotates right. In the non-neutral positions, when you sidebend right, your vertebra rotates right and when you sidebend left, your vertebra rotates left. When sidebending and rotation are coupled to opposite sides it is called Type I motion and when they are coupled to the same sides it is called Type II motion. This classification of spinal motion into Type I and Type II is a description of normal motion. Dysfunction arises only if there is some sort of restriction or facet fixation involved.

An important point to remember is that sidebending and rotation always happen together along the spine. A vertebra or group of vertebrae can never rotate without also sidebending and never sidebend without also rotating. Interestingly, the lumbar spine can sidebend more than it can rotate and the thoracic spine can rotate more than it can sidebend. The cervical spine behaves differently from the lumbar and thoracic spines in one very important respect: regardless of whether you forward or backward bend, the motion of C2–C7 is always Type II. The neck is different enough from the thoracic and lumbar spines that it deserves its own chapter. So for the remainder of this chapter and through the next couple of chapters we will be discussing only the thoracic and lumbar spines.

Since we will be using rotation as our starting point for determining and treating facet dysfunction, let's explore palpating vertebral rotation a bit more. If you are a soft-tissue practitioner and you haven't assessed vertebral rotation before, your highly developed palpatory skills for assessing soft tissue strain and tightness may mislead you in your first attempts to feel bone. If you are like many soft-tissue practitioners I have taught, when you try to get a sense of the tissue beneath your fingers, you often gently niggle it—you poke a bit here and prod a bit there—often you move your fingers up and down, back and forth, and in small circles. But when you feel for bone, you must resist the temptation to palpate in this way. Instead, you should apply gentle but firm and constant pressure as you let your fingers sink into the tissue until they come to an obvious stopping point where they can sink no further. When they can sink no further and you feel a hard stopping point, you have reached bone. This hard stopping point feels different than tight or strained soft tissue.

Imagine that a vertebra you are palpating is right rotated. As your thumbs sink through the tissue and come to rest on the bony surface of the vertebra, you will notice that your right thumb stops sinking into the tissue before the left thumb does. To say it differently, you will notice that your right thumb has come to rest on a bony bump that is a little more posterior and prominent than where the left thumb landed. Your left thumb in contrast seems to have sunk into a little indentation and is hence a little more anterior than the right thumb. If you niggle the tissue as you are letting your thumbs sink toward the vertebra, you can easily get confused about what you are feeling.

Ask one of your friends or clients to volunteer his back and sit comfortably straight in the neutral position. Keep your thumbs in the same horizontal plane facing each other, each just slightly lateral to the spinous processes of the vertebra you are palpating. Make sure that the palmer surfaces of your thumbs cover the transverse processes. Keeping your thumbs in this horizontal position, run them up and down your friend's thoracic spine until you find a vertebra with one transverse process that is obviously more posterior or prominent than the others (Figures 1.3 and 1.4, page 6). Don't worry about those vertebrae that you are not sure about—ignore them for now and only look for the most obvious ones. Once you find a transverse process that is obviously more prominent or posterior on one side, you have found a rotated vertebra. The vertebra is rotated to the side where you feel the prominent transverse process. The

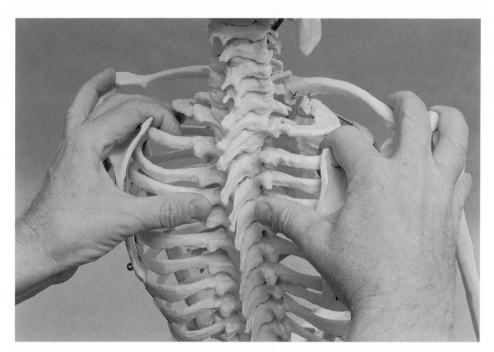

Figure 1.3

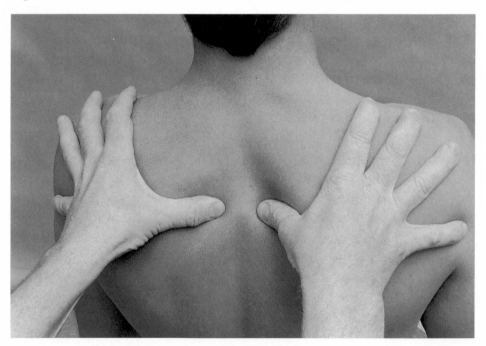

Figure 1.4

easy way to remember how to designate rotation is to remember that the *side of the bump is the side of the rotation*. If you feel the bump on the left (with an indentation on the right), the vertebra is left-rotated. If you feel the bump on the right (with an indentation on the left), the vertebra is right-rotated.

To be more precise in your description, you should follow the convention and designate the rotation you feel in reference to the next vertebra just below it. This convention makes good sense because what you are ultimately interested in understanding is joint fixation and you cannot have a joint, let alone a fixated one, without two contiguous bones. So if you find that T7 is right-rotated, you would say that T7 is rotated right on T8. You can say it any reasonable way you want to, of course, and there are many different conventions for designating rotation. But I have adopted the conventions of the osteopaths, because they constantly scrutinize their language for consistency and accuracy. I should mention that even though I use descriptive conventions derived from osteopathy, I do not discuss or borrow their techniques for this book. Unless otherwise noted, all the techniques you will learn in this book were my own creation and are soft-tissue techniques, not high-velocity, low-amplitude osseous manipulations.

Experiment with feeling for rotation with a lot of different backs and always begin with the most obvious rotations along the thoracic spine first. On the whole it is much easier to feel rotations of the thoracic spine in a sitting position than it is to feel them in the lumbar spine. Above all, don't fret about the vertebrae whose rotational patterns are not clear to your fingers. As you gain confidence in feeling for the obvious cases, in time you will also gain sensitivity in feeling for the less obvious ones.

After you gain some confidence with the thoracic spine, try feeling for rotations in the lumbar spine. First feel for rotation in the sitting position. Then ask your volunteer to lie prone on your treatment table and feel the same areas in this position. In the sitting position the erectors are working to maintain an upright posture and since many people's back muscles are overdeveloped, you will find that it is often difficult to feel through these muscles to the bone beneath. In the prone position you will find it is much easier to feel the transverse processes through the back muscles.

In order to better determine which vertebrae you are palpating you need a few landmarks from which to take your bearings. If you trace a hor-

7

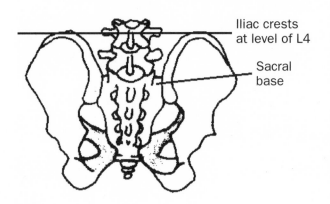

Iliac crests
at level of L4

Sacral
base

Figure 1.5

izontal line across from the crest of the ilium to the spine, your fingers will land the spinous process of L4 (Figure 1.5). From there you can count down one spinous process to find L5 or up to determine L3, L2, and L1.

To find T1 place your fingers on your best guess to locate C6 and ask your volunteer to bend his head and neck backward. If you are on C6 as your volunteer bends, it will slide obviously anteriorly. If you are on C7 it will not move in this way at all. If you don't have a volunteer as you read this, you can try it on yourself. Once you have located C6 you can easily count down spinous processes to find T1, T2, and so forth. This test for anterior sliding of C6 with back bending works quite well most of the time for most people. But be forewarned: on occasion you will find a person whose cervicothoracic junction is fixated in a way that makes this test useless.

Another useful landmark for finding your way through the spine is the inferior tip of the scapula. If you trace a horizontal line from the inferior tip to the spine, your fingers will most likely land around T8.

A Simple Indirect Technique

NOW THAT YOU HAVE SOME EXPERIENCE PALPATING ROTATION, WE CAN build on your knowledge by practicing a simple, indirect technique for derotating vertebrae. This technique was discovered by a number of therapists independently of each other. Ask your volunteer to sit comfortably. Find the most obviously rotated vertebra in his thoracic spine. For the purpose of this discussion, let's assume that you find that T4 is right rotated on T5. What you will feel is your right thumb resting on the bump (the prominent, posterior transverse process of T4) and your left

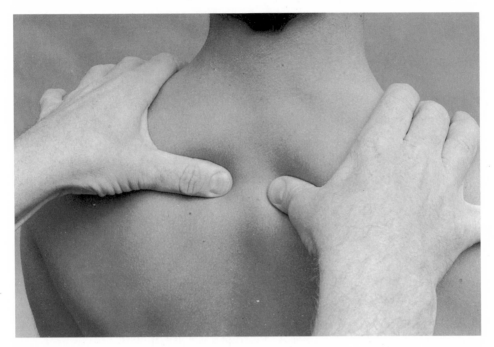

Figure 1.6

thumb resting in an indentation (the anterior transverse process of T4).

To begin the technique, use your left thumb to apply a couple of pounds of gentle but firm pressure to the left transverse process (TP) with the intention of making it sink more anteriorly (Figure 1.6). If you are not used to this sort of technique, the idea of pushing the anterior TP more anteriorly may seem counter-intuitive and a bit odd. You might be thinking that it would make more mechanical sense to push the right posterior TP anteriorly as a way to derotate it. But bodies are not machines and they have profoundly interesting ways of responding to intelligent pressure that will make your life as a somatic practitioner easier than you might imagine. This is called an indirect technique because it does not directly force change on the spine the way high-velocity, low-amplitude thrusting techniques do. Indirect techniques begin by pushing a dysfunctional segment further into its dysfunction and letting it wind its way back to where a normal position is. Don't worry about why this technique works. Just enjoy how your volunteer's body responds to pushing the left anterior TP more anteriorly.

When you apply your pressure to the left TP of T4, imagine that you are pushing a boat away from a dock. If you push too quickly and too hard, you will experience resistance. But if you push in a slow, gentle, firm way, the boat will almost effortlessly drift away from the dock. As you first push anteriorly on the left TP, nothing happens for a few seconds. But notice that as you keep the pressure up, your left thumb begins to sink a little more anteriorly as your right thumb begins to move a little more posteriorly. You are actually feeling T4 go further into right rotation. You may even feel it go into sidebending. Maintain the image of pushing a boat away from a dock in the back of your mind, and keep the pressure up, but don't force the issue; just push and continue to follow this motion until it stops. Before it stops the vertebra may rotate and sidebend in odd and unpredictable ways. Don't worry about it or question it, just follow the motion until it stops.

At that point, T4 will have moved as far it can go into right rotation. There will be a pause, sometimes accompanied by the feeling of a little pulsation under your thumbs. Just wait and soon you will feel the impulse of the vertebra to start derotating as if it were moving into left rotation. You may feel it sidebend and rotate left, then right, and in other odd and unpredictable ways before it finally stops, but stay with it. It will stop moving when it is derotated and when it stops you will also feel a softening of the tissues under your thumbs. If you wait a little longer you may also feel the spine lengthening above and/or below your thumbs, as if the body were organizing itself along vertical lines in response to the release of the vertebra. When you feel the tissue softening and sense the body organizing itself along the sagittal plane you are finished. If you don't feel the body organizing itself along this line, don't worry about it—as long as your thumbs remain in contact with the body, it will organize itself around the release whether you feel it or not. Just wait for the softening and then wait just a bit longer afterward. If you use this technique with the expectation of feeling that you can sense how the body organizes itself around the vertical release, in time you will actually sense this orthotropic effect.

Being able to feel how the body organizes or fails to organize itself in relation to your intervention is a very useful skill to learn and it will allow you to tell immediately what other areas body require intervention. Interestingly, not only does the body organize itself around the sagittal plane, it also organizes itself simultaneously around the transverse and coronal planes. Knowing how to feel for the presence or absence of this orthogonal relationship tells you when you are finished with your technique and where to go next.

The simple technique you have just learned will open many interesting doorways for you if you just keep practicing it and feeling for as much information as you can. But this indirect technique, like so many indirect techniques (or so-called "unwinding techniques"), is not always effective. You will notice that sometimes you will achieve easy and amazing results with it and at other times the problem you thought you had taken care of reasserts itself within a matter of minutes or hours. The drawback with most unwinding techniques is that they often do not address one of the most important aspects of a painful back—the underlying facet restriction. Most indirect techniques tend to unwind the tissues and vertebra around the joint fixation. Since the joint fixation has not been resolved, the problem quickly returns. To deal with the facet restriction, you first need to understand how facet fixations work and then you need a soft-tissue technique that challenges the joint fixation. This is what you will learn in the next two chapters.

CHAPTER

2

Primates in Trouble, or where does your back go when it goes out?

HOW MANY TIMES HAVE YOU HEARD THIS SURPRISED COMMENT FROM a client? "You know, I was just bending over to pick up something, when all of a sudden I felt something slip in my lower back and the next thing I know I'm on my knees in terrible pain!"

There are many levels to, and competing explanations for, how the spine becomes compromised. The important point is that facets not only get engaged in forward bending and sidebending, they sometimes escalate an already strained relationship into a bad marriage and remain severely fixated. When we forward bend or back bend and then twist (sidebend), we put our low backs at risk. If you were to examine your client's unhappy marriage when he is in the neutral position (sitting or standing comfortably straight), you would discover that one or more of his lumbar vertebra is stuck so that it is sidebent and rotated to the same side. In neutral position, thoracic and lumbar vertebrae are not supposed to act this way. So if you find a vertebra in neutral position that is stuck rotated and sidebent to the same side, you are probably looking at a person in pain.

At this point you may be thinking, "Wait a minute, if, as you say, it is much easier to feel rotation than sidebending, how can you know whether a vertebra is rotated to the same or opposite side of the sidebending?" The answer is simple: every time you find a vertebra in neutral position that is stuck sidebent and rotated to the same side, you have discovered restricted facets. Because the facets are restricted, there is loss of normal motion in the area. If facets are fixed, the vertebra will not be able to move normally in back bending and forward bending. The restricted facets will act as fixed pivot points that will force the vertebra to move in characteristically errant ways as your client bends forward and backward. By feeling how the vertebra rotates around this fixed pivot point in forward and back bending you will be able to determine precisely which facets are restricted and how they are restricted. Once you know this, treating them is easy and obvious.

But before we consider the facet-restriction test, let's deal with a very important clinical question: where does your back go when it goes out? This is one of those odd questions like "Where does your lap go when you stand up?" or "Where does fire go when it goes out?" that seems as though it should have an answer, but doesn't. These sorts of questions don't have answers not because they are too difficult for anyone to answer, but because they are confused questions.

I stated the question this way to make an important point about the nature of spinal dysfunction. Somatic therapists and non-therapists alike tend to describe back pain by saying, "Your back is out." But this expression is imprecise and even quite misleading. The critical point is not that a client's back "went out," as if its new position were the primary problem, but that there are facet restrictions and loss of function associated with the client's pain. Treatment consists not of putting it back where it belongs, but in releasing the restricted facets in order to restore function. Where the vertebra goes after you release it from its facet restrictions is sometimes quite different for each person. Along the same lines, if you were able to get the vertebra to "go back to where it belongs" (derotate it) and you didn't release the restricted facets, the person's back would still be dysfunctional and it would not be long until the pain returned. If you have been experimenting with the simple indirect technique introduced in the last chapter, you already know that it is not always effective. Now you know why.

Some vertebral dysfunctions also have very little to do with the position of the vertebrae. For example, often the facets on both sides of the spine can be restricted, but the vertebra shows no obvious palpatable signs of being "out of place" (rotated and sidebent). When both sides are restricted, your client will have pain and loss of motion in the area. Again,

14

the treatment goal is to release the facet restrictions so that you can restore proper functioning, not reposition vertebrae. Many times you will find vertebrae that are rotated and still perfectly functional because no facet or myofascial restrictions are interfering with motion in the area. Given the unique structure of that person in relation to how his body has adapted to gravity and the stresses of life, his vertebrae probably can only be right where they are. They are not likely to be functional in any other position. If you had the power to force his vertebrae into some version of the ideal position, you would probably just create pain for him.

In order to more clearly understand the role of joint manipulation and the role of positioning body structure and segments, it is very helpful to preview the words of physiologist I.M. Korr. Discussing the non-segmented "symphonies" of motor activity that are orchestrated and carried out by the spinal cord and higher centers, he says:

> The important point is that these patterns of activity involve neurons up and down the spinal cord, each being called into play according to the pattern required at the moment—not according to where the neuron is located in the cord but according to what structure it innervates. Where it "lives" segmentally is of no importance ...
>
> This presents us with an interesting paradox: the normal patterns of activity mediated by the spinal cord are completely non-segmental in nature ... yet the spinal cord is obviously segmented and the physician is very much concerned with segmental relationships.... Nevertheless, in normal life segmental relationships do not appear.
>
> The reason for this paradox may be best conveyed by [an] illustrative simile. Consider a beautifully executed parade of skilled marching men, where the many ranks and columns are seen as patterned activity of the whole parade. We do not see individual ranks and certainly not individual marchers, we see patterned motion. But let something go wrong, let one of the marchers lose step and his rank immediately becomes conspicuous. The other marchers cannot compensate in a coordinated manner and soon the ranks on either side are thrown into confusion and then we

15

do see segmental relationship. It is something like this that causes segmental relationships in the spine to emerge into view.... A segment "in view" is a segment in trouble....

How shall we reconcile this paradox? First by realizing that the thing that is segmented is the armor that houses and protects the cord.... In normal life the segmentation is not of the spinal cord itself; the segmentation is in the assembling of the nerve fibers into "cables"—roots and nerves—that can pass out to the tissues innervated. What is segmented is ingress and egress, not the *function* of the cord itself.[1]

We can see even more clearly from Dr. Korr's wonderful example of the marchers how spinal manipulation is not a simple matter of repositioning or putting bones "back into place." The ultimate aim of spinal manipulation is the recovery of normal patterned motion, not the creation of an ideal position for the segments. By implication, the aim is also not the creation of a spine that measures up to some ideal pattern. When a vertebral segment or a group of vertebrae become "segments in view," to use Dr. Korr's phrase, we perceive a loss of patterned motion throughout the spine. Part of what we see are breaks or fixations in the overall continuity of structure and movement. We see loss of continuity and appropriate motion. The "segments in view" often show up as fixations in the myofascial, ligamentous, and articular systems. These fixations create varying degrees of local immobility, which in turn inhibit normal integrated movement throughout the whole body.

With this new understanding, let's reconsider those people whose backs "went out" when they bent over. All of them were well on their way to having back problems before they first experienced back pain. Think of what happens when you put water on the stove to boil. You turn up the heat and the water gets hotter and hotter. Suddenly it passes a certain temperature threshold and boils. If the water were conscious, the first time it was brought to a boil it might say, "You know it was really weird, I was just hanging out on the stove feeling the heat when all of sudden I began to boil!" Analogously your clients' backs were "heating up" to "go out."

Myofascial, ligamentous, and facet restrictions were already present; there were larger overall patterns of imbalance in their bodies; their legs

16

probably were not providing adequate support; there were dysfunctional adaptations to old injuries and to gravity; and vertebrae were slightly more toward a Type II position than was good for them. Then the fatal day arrived when your client passed his critical threshold by bending over and slightly twisting (sidebending) to pick something up. During this movement, his vertebra slipped a little too quickly and a little too far past what was normal for a Type II position. The nervous system registered the danger and sent the muscles into a fearful spasm thereby locking the vertebra into a Type II position and creating facet restrictions. There are other ways you can lock up your back, of course, but this simple case is useful because it allows us to understand how facets become restricted. The important point is that facet fixations create a motion restriction that adversely affects the way the rest of the spine behaves in walking and other forms of movement. And over time it can facilitate other facet restrictions.

If your spine has no facet restrictions, when you forward bend, your facets slide open in an accordion-like fashion and when you back bend they slide closed. As you forward bend, each vertebra in relation to the one inferior to it slides slightly superiorly and anteriorly. When you back bend the opposite occurs: each vertebra slides slightly inferiorly and posteriorly.

Now, if facets are restricted, they will act as a fixed point around which the vertebra will be forced to rotate when you forward and back bend. The side on which the facets are restricted remains fixed during forward and backward bending, while the other side appears to rotate and derotate. To say it differently, one side of the vertebra remains a fixed pivot point around which the other side moves anteriorly and posteriorly in forward and backward bending, respectively.

Figures 2.1 and 2.2, page 18, show rather clearly the effects of forward bending and backward bending on the behavior of the facets. During back bending the facets slide toward a closed position and during forward bending they slide toward an open position.

Figure 2.3 shows a dysfunctional vertebra. What you are looking at are two vertebrae in neutral position. The superior vertebra is stuck right rotated and right sidebent. Notice how the facets on the left have slid open and the facets on the right have slid closed. Since we are looking at a Type II dysfunction, one side must be restricted. Either the left facets are fixed open (in flexion or forward bending) or the right facets are fixed closed

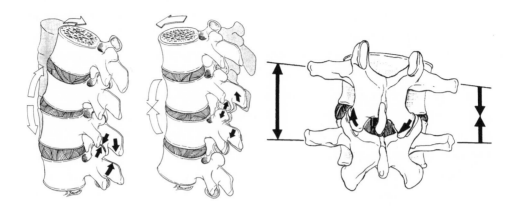

Figure 2.1   *Figure 2.2*   *Figure 2.3*

(in extension or backward bending). But which facets are fixed?

Remember that restricted facets create a fixed pivot point around which the vertebra is forced to rotate in forward and backward bending. So if you were to place your thumbs on the transverse processes of the superior vertebra and feel for how it rotates and derotates during forward and backward bending, you could determine which facets were fixed. You would know whether the left facets were fixed open or the right facets were fixed closed. And once you knew which and how the facets were restricted, you could simply and easily release them.

But before you learn how to apply the test, let's explore a technique for releasing facet restrictions first. For many somatic therapists, learning a simple facet release technique that doesn't require precise knowledge of which facet is fixed is the best way to deepen their palpatory and conceptual understanding of how to apply the test. Many hands-on therapists find that if they can get this understanding into their hands first, they have an easier time getting it into their heads. The technique you are about to learn is a kind of shotgun approach to a more specific way to address facet restrictions. From the clinical standpoint, this approach is less efficient than the one you will use once you know how to apply the test. But from the learning standpoint this approach is a far more effective teaching technique. You will also be happy to know that it is, for the most part, as effective as the more efficient approach.

When you find a rotated vertebra, just pretend that it is a Type II fixation. It may turn out, of course, that the rotated vertebra you picked is not dysfunctional at all. If it isn't stuck rotated and sidebent to the same side when in the neutral position and you apply this shotgun approach, the worst thing that will happen is that you will have wasted your time (and your client's). Since rotated vertebrae with restricted facets are more common than flowers in the Spring, the best thing that will happen is that you will actually put your finger on the source of your client's pain and by applying this technique release her from her misery.

If the rotated vertebra you pick is sidebent and rotated to the same side in the neutral position, it will have restricted facets and it will be a dysfunctional Type II. And this is always true: either the facets are fixed closed on the side of the prominent or posterior TP (the same side to which it is rotated) or they are fixed open opposite to the side of the prominent TP (opposite to the side to which it is rotated).

The technique for releasing fixed open or fixed closed facets is simple. Since you don't know which facets are restricted, you simply treat both sides as if they were fixed. Let's say that you found T3 is right rotated on T4. If the problem is with the right facets, it is because they are fixed closed and cannot open in forward bending. If the problem is with the left facets, they are fixed open and cannot close in back bending. Pick the right facets first. If your client is sitting, ask him to curl over into a forward bent position. Put a knuckle or elbow in the right spinal groove on the presumed fixed closed facets (Figures 2.4 and 2.5, page 20). Slowly and firmly apply 5 to 10 pounds of continuous pressure to the facets and let your knuckle or elbow sink to where it can go no further. Wait until you feel the tissue soften and give way under your pressure. (See if you can also feel the orthotropic effect as the body lengthens and organizes itself along the sagittal plane after the facets release.) Then return your client to a neutral sitting position. Put your knuckle or elbow in the left spinal groove on the facets that are presumed fixed open. Instruct your client to back bend while you slowly and firmly apply 5 to 10 pounds of pressure (Figure 2.6, page 21). Let your knuckle or elbow sink to where it can sink no further and wait until you feel the tissue soften and give way under your pressure. (Again, see if you can feel the orthotropic effect as the body lengthens and organizes itself along the sagittal plane after the facets

19

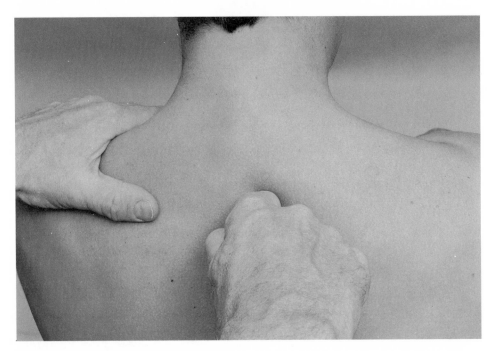

Figure 2.4

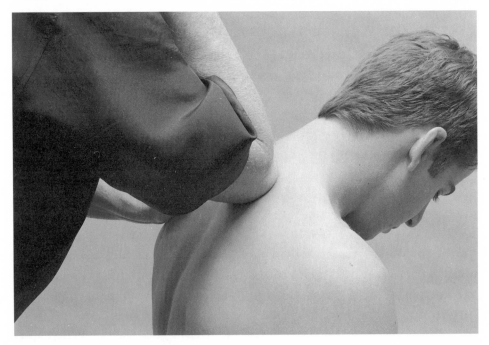

Figure 2.5

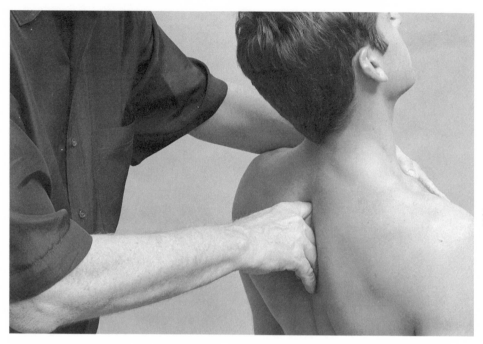

Figure 2.6

release.) After you have applied this technique to both sides, check T3 to make sure that it is no longer rotated.

Whether you are releasing fixed closed or fixed open facets, as long as you keep the pressure up (just waiting for the softening, the sense of the tissue giving way, and the spine lengthening and organizing itself along the sagittal plane) it is enough to release the facets. With time and practice you may begin to feel the facets actually close or open, but it is not necessary for you to feel the facets release for the technique to work. As you learn to feel the facets release, you will also begin to feel a corollary phenomenon, namely that not much happens under your fingers when you apply pressure to unrestricted facets. In time you want to be able to feel the facets release, the tissue soften, and the body lengthen and organize itself along the sagittal plane. Although tenderness or pain is not always the best evaluative tool, you will often find that the soft tissues associated with the problematic facets is tender or painful when you apply pressure.

Practice this shotgun technique on the thoracic vertebrae first with your client in a sitting position. Then practice it with the lumbar verte-

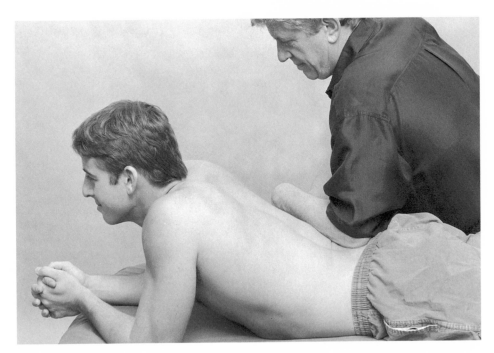

Figure 2.7

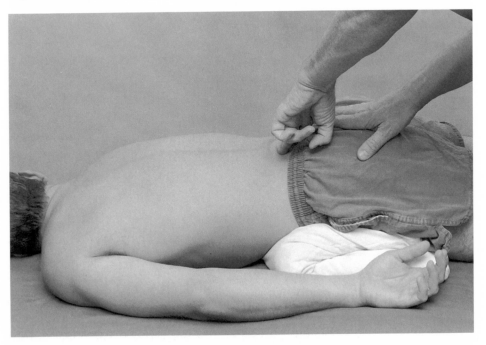

Figure 2.8

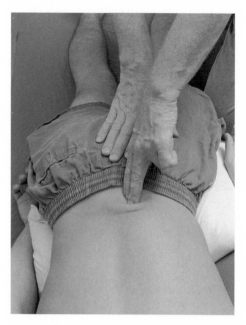

Figure 2.9

brae. Until you are more confident in your ability to feel rotation in the lumbar vertebrae, always check what you feel in the sitting position against what you feel in the prone position. Once you are sure that a lumbar vertebra is rotated, you can use the sitting position to release facet restrictions in much the same way you learned to release the thoracic vertebrae.

You can also release lumbar facet restrictions with your client prone. Suppose you find that L5 is left rotated. Begin with the assumption that the right facets are fixed open. Instruct your client to raise himself up on his elbows and to rest in that position. Then apply pressure to the right side of the spinal groove where the presumed fixed open facets are and wait for them to release (Figure 2.7). Then double over a pillow and place it under your client's abdomen so that the lumbar spine is appropriately flexed. Apply pressure to the left side where the presumed fixed closed facets are and wait for them to release (Figures 2.8 and 2.9).

The side-lying position is also a very effective way to release facet restrictions in both lumbar and thoracic vertebrae. To release presumed fixed-closed facets, instruct your client to lie in a tight fetal position on the side of his body opposite the closed facets. Apply pressure with your knuckle or elbow to the facets and wait for them to release (Figures 2.10, 2.11, and 2.12, pages 24 and 25). Ask him to roll over on his other side and back bend as you apply pressure to the presumed fixed open facets and wait for them to release (Figure 2.12).

It will make your life as a manual therapist just a little easier if you understand something about how the thoracic facets of the spine are arranged: parallel to the coronal plane. You can use this arrangement to your advantage. When you are releasing closed thoracic facets you will be

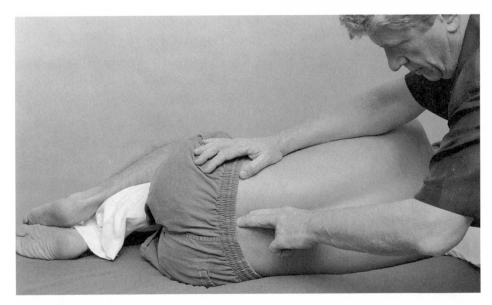

Figure 2.10

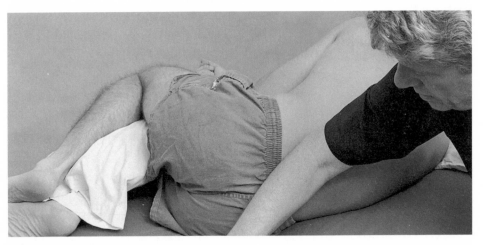

Figure 2.11

slightly more effective and efficient if you apply pressure in a cephalad direction. With open-fixed thoracic facets, the technique will work just a little bit better if you apply pressure in a caudad direction. The lumbar and cervical facets are clearly not arranged in the same way as the thoracic facets, so the direction in which you apply pressure is not as important.

As you practice this technique you will quickly understand why it is more

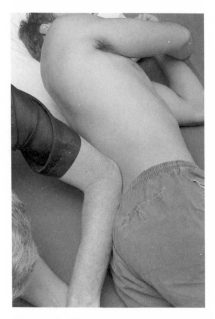

Figure 2.12

effective than the indirect technique introduced in the last chapter. The problem with the indirect technique is that it doesn't address the fixed facets, whereas this new technique actually challenges the facet restrictions. If the facets are fixed closed the technique requires that you put your client in a forward-bent position to encourage the facets to open while you release the tissues responsible for the restriction. In the same way, when the facets are fixed open, back bending encourages the facets to close as you release the restricting tissues. The indirect technique is probably only successful when the restrictions are not very severe. Generally speaking, if you want to release a joint anywhere in the body, it is almost always more effective to use a technique that challenges the restricted facets rather than a technique that simply unwinds tissue around the fixation.

Keep practicing this shotgun approach until you gain confidence with feeling rotation and releasing facet restrictions. In the next chapter, you will learn how to apply the test so you don't waste time trying to release what is not restricted.

Note

1. Korr, I.M. "Vulnerability of the Segmental Nervous System to Somatic Insults" in *The Physiological Basis of Osteopathic Medicine*, George W. Northup ed., (New York, 1982), pp 56–57. Emphasis added.

CHAPTER

3

Finding and Fixing the Fixations

WHENEVER YOU ARE LOOKING AT A VERTEBRA THAT IS ROTATED and sidebent to the same side (Type II), whether it is dysfunctional or normal, the facets on the side with the prominent TP (the side to which it is rotated) are always closed and the opposite facets are open. If all is normal and no facets are restricted, normal motion is possible through the area. If the situation is dysfunctional, there are restricted facets and an obvious loss of motion. So when you find a rotation, you need a way to determine which facets are restricted so you don't waste time trying to release facets that are not restricted. If you find restricted facets in the lumbar or thoracic spine, then they are either fixed open or fixed closed. Again, you need a way to determine whether the open facets are fixed or the closed facets are fixed to avoid wasting time. The cervical facets are unlike the thoracic and lumbar facets in that one side can be fixed open while the other is fixed closed. If C3 is right-rotated and right sidebent on C4, it is possible for the right facets to be fixed closed and the left facets to be fixed open. But this kind of bilateral fixation does not occur in the thoracic and lumbar facets. For now we are only going to deal with the lumbar and thoracic facets. In the next chapter we will examine the cervical facets.

The test for determining which thoracic or lumbar facets are restricted and how they are restricted is fairly easy to perform, but somewhat complicated to explain, although there is a very simple way to remember the

27

important information you can gather from it.

With your client in a sitting position, find the most obviously rotated thoracic vertebra. Say you find that T3 is right rotated on T4 and let's assume that the left facets are the restricted ones. Since they are fixed open, in a position of flexion or forward bending, when your client bends forward the left TP remains stationary, fixed slightly anteriorly. Meanwhile, your right thumb will follow the right TP as it moves anteriorly during forward bending. The right TP moves anteriorly during forward bending, because that is what it does normally. But because the left side is already fixed anteriorly, the right TP is forced to pivot around the open-fixed left facet as your client bends forward. As a result, the right side appears to derotate. To say it differently, when your client forward bends, the bump on the right seems to disappear and the indentation on the left stays where it is (Figure 3.1). When your client returns to neutral position, the bump on the right reappears. If your client now back bends, the bump on the right will appear to get more extreme and the vertebra will move more into right rotation (Figure 3.2). As your client back bends the fixed pivot point created by left facets keeps the left TP fixed anteriorly. Since back bending forces the right side to move more posteriorly in comparison to the fixed indentation on the left, the right TP appears to move further into right rotation.

Now let's imagine the opposite situation in which the right side is fixed closed, as if the right facets were backward bent (or extended). As a result, the right TP will be fixed posteriorly. When your client back bends, your thumbs feel the vertebra derotate and the bump seems to go away. Why? Because the right TP is already fixed posteriorly and the left TP is forced to pivot around the fixed right facets and move posteriorly as your client back bends. Since the left side is free to move posteriorly and the right side is fixed posteriorly already, back bending removes the indentation as the left TP moves posteriorly to match the right TP. When your client returns to neutral, the bump on the right returns. If your client now forward bends, the bump seems to become more extreme. Since the right facets are fixed closed, the right TP is fixed posteriorly. Since the left facets are free, as your client forward bends they allow the left TP to move anteriorly in comparison to the right TP which is fixed posteriorly. The difference between the two TP's is now more extreme and your thumbs seem

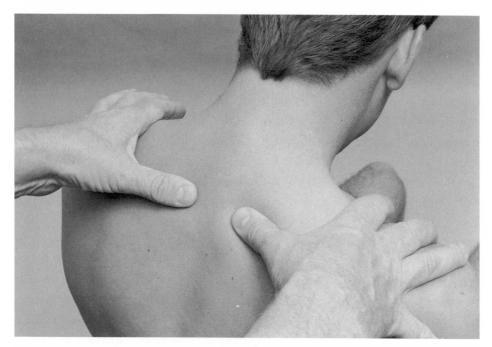

Figure 3.1

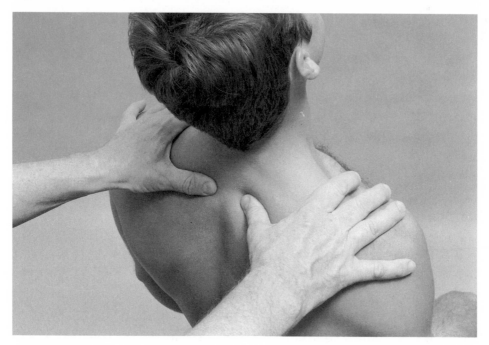

Figure 3.2

to sense that the vertebra has moved into a more extreme right rotation.

The preceding procedure is the basis of the test for determining rotation and sidebending, and identifying which facets are restricted. But let me caution you about a very important point: if you are like most other practitioners who are new to this test, you will probably try to think your way through what happens each time you perform the test. As your client forward and backward bends, you will be tempted to describe to yourself what you are feeling, similar to the way I just described it. Don't do it, because there is an easy way to remember the information for identifying which facet to release. Describing to yourself a complicated phenomenon (that also demands that you deduce the side on which the facets are restricted from the way a vertebra rotates and derotates during forward and backward bending as you remember that it is sidebent and rotated to the same side) while simultaneously trying to feel what is happening under your thumbs for the first time in your life is 100 times more difficult than trying to follow this awkward sentence I am writing trying to describe what you shouldn't attempt. What you need is a simple rule that will allow you to identify and treat the facet fixation with palpatory ease and very little conceptual thought.

First you determine rotation in neutral position. Keep your thumbs on the TP's of the rotated vertebra, forward and backward bend your client, and feel and watch what happens under your thumbs. Look for the position (whether in forward or backward bending) where the bump (the posterior or prominent TP of the rotated vertebra) disappears. Some people object to saying the bump disappears and like to say that the vertebra appears to derotate. This is a matter of taste, so use whatever description works best. But remember this important point: *the position where the bump disappears (or the vertebra appears to derotate) is the position in which the facets are restricted.* If the bump disappears in forward bending, the facets are fixed in the forward bent position, which means the facets are fixed open (flexion fixed). If the bump disappears in back bending, the facets are fixed in the back bent position, which means the facets are fixed closed (extension fixed).

There is one more important reminder: if the bump, or posterior TP, disappears in forward bending, the fixed-open facets are on the opposite side of the rotation, or posterior TP. If the bump disappears in back bending, the fixed-closed facets are on the same side of the rotation. In other words, if a vertebra in neutral position is rotated and sidebent to the same side (Type II dysfunction), it has a facet restriction and the facets are either fixed open or fixed closed. If they are fixed closed, the fixed facets are on the same side as the rotation, or posterior TP. If they are fixed open, the fixed facets are on the opposite side of the rotation, or prominent TP.

So here are two very simple rules that will allow you to keep your sanity as you practice this test:

In *backward bending* if the prominent TP disappears,
the facets on the side of the rotation are *fixed closed.*

In *forward bending* if the prominent TP disappears,
the facets on the side opposite to the rotation are *fixed open.*

You can reformulate these rules any way you want, but keep a copy of them where you can easily see them as you practice performing the test. Again, don't try to think through the logic of this test as you perform it. Learn how to apply the test and get the information you need by using these rules first. In time, if it is important to you to be able to state the logic of the test to yourself or to others, you can practice doing it. For now, use this easy method to determine whether the facets are restricted and whether they are fixed open or closed so that you can directly and effortlessly release them.

The techniques for releasing facet restrictions are the same as those you learned in the last chapter. Since you now have a quick way to determine whether you are dealing with fixed open or fixed closed facets, you only need to apply the technique to the side with the facet restriction. So if the facets are fixed open, apply the technique in any of the back bending positions (sitting, prone, or sidelying). If the facets are fixed closed, apply the technique in any of the forward bending positions.

Previously I mentioned that facets can be bilaterally fixed open or closed. These fixations are not as easy to find through palpation because they do not show up as rotated and sidebent. Test for them by putting your client in the sitting position. Find the suspected vertebrae and put a finger or thumb on the spinous process of the superior vertebra and put the finger or thumb of the other hand on the spinous process immediately inferior, and instruct your client to bend forward and backward (Figures 3.3 and

31

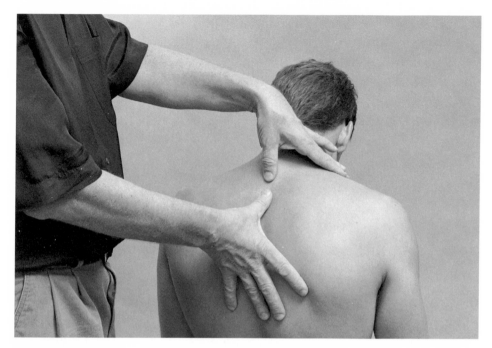

Figure 3.3

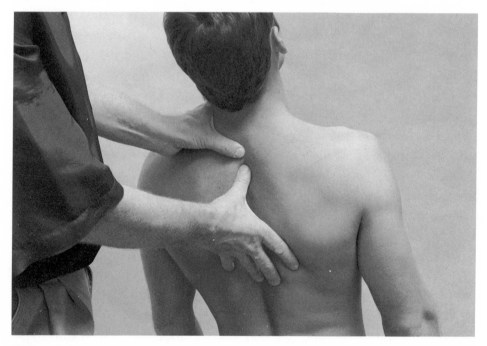

Figure 3.4

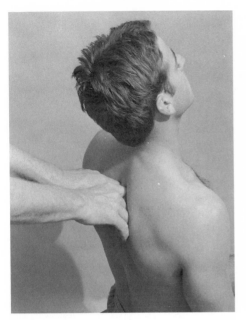

Figure 3.5

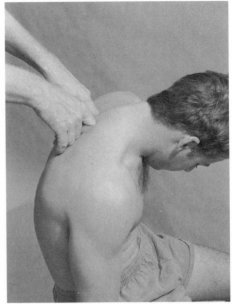

Figure 3.6

3.4). If your thumbs move away from each other in forward bending, but do not approximate in backward bending, the facets are bilaterally fixed open. If your thumbs approximate in backward bending, but do not move apart in forward bending, the facets are bilaterally fixed closed.

Releasing either is quite simple. Again with your client in the sitting position, place the knuckle of your right forefinger in the right spinal groove and the knuckle of your left forefinger in the left spinal groove. If the facets are bilaterally fixed open, ask your client to back bend over your knuckles as you apply pressure to both sides and wait for the release (Figure 3.5). If the facets are bilaterally fixed closed, ask your client to forward bend, apply pressure to both facets, and wait for the release (Figure 3.6). You can apply these techniques in the prone or sidelying positions if you wish, but for obvious reasons you will probably find the sitting position the easiest and most efficient.

As you practice the test for unilateral facet restrictions, you will find vertebrae that are obviously rotated, but do not respond to forward and backward bending by appearing to rotate and derotate. You will probably also notice that these vertebrae often group themselves together into a curva-

33

ture. What you are looking at are Type I group fixations. When you forward and backward bend clients with group fixations, the rotated vertebrae stay in their rotated position all the way through the process of forward and backward bending. If, as is often the case, they are a part of a rotoscoliosis (Figure 3.7), their positions are fixed because of larger myofascial restrictions and because the shape of the vertebrae has been altered as part of the curvature. Type I dysfunctions tend not to be restricted at the facet level by the small muscles and the ligaments like Type II dysfunctions are.

You should be aware that within a Type I curvature you can find individual dysfunctional Type II vertebrae. As you might imagine, they are a little hard to find. Suppose your client's thoracic vertebrae are all right sidebent and left rotated, except for one. That one vertebra could be left rotated and left sidebent or right rotated and right sidebent. If it is rotated right and sidebent right it will be nearly impossible to differentiate it from the other vertebrae that are also right rotated by feel alone. If it is left rotated and left sidebent, since it is also shaped in the Type I pattern, it will still be very difficult to differentiate. You can find it if you apply the forward/backward bending test. But realize that it is also part of the curvature, so don't expect it to appear to derotate all the way. Since one of the facets is restricted, it will appear to rotate and derotate to some degree. And it is that degree of rotating and derotating you have to get a feel for if you want to locate Type II dysfunctions in the midst of Type I patterns.

In any case, if you find some vertebrae in thoracic or lumbar spine that do not change how they are rotated in forward and backward bending, they are Type I fixations. They require a slightly more complicated technique than what you have learned so far and you will learn these techniques in Chapter Ten.

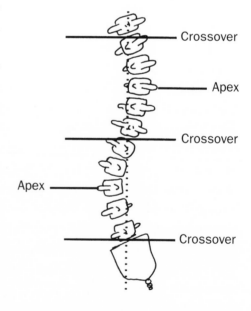

Figure 3.7

CHAPTER

4

The Neck

I N HIS MONUMENTAL WORK, *The Interpretation of Dreams,* FREUD SAID THAT the royal road to the unconscious is through dream interpretation. His brilliant colleague, Wilhelm Reich, said that the royal road is through understanding the body. Well, after many years of working with people in various kinds of distress, I have come to see that they are both wrong— it's the neck!

Of course, my claim is an exaggeration. But like all such exaggerations it contains some degree of truth. The cervical vertebrae support a rather large and heavy egg shaped thing that is constantly moving about, sticking a fleshy protuberance called a nose into situations that often don't concern it. Our emotions often begin their journey toward expression in our bellies and wind their way through our neck—one of the major thoroughfares through which they eventually get expressed. If we suppress our emotions, we often do it by tightening the complicated musculature of the neck. If we do this over a long enough period of time, we can lose a good deal of our flexibility and create a rather painful bottleneck. Also, since the cervical spine is not embedded as securely in bony, myofascial, membranous structures as the thoracic and lumbar spines, it can move in many interesting and complicated ways—and as a result get into trouble more easily. Since the neck is so highly flexible, it is better able to adapt to imbalances in the rest of the body than other parts of the spine.

Try standing up and sidebending to the right. Notice how your shoulder girdle and neck respond. You would actually be more comfortable if your neck followed the sidebending. But because of your righting reflexes you instinctively look ahead with your eyes roughly horizontal to the ground plane. Notice how your neck loses some of its flexibility as you attempt to keep your head on straight while sidebending. In a less exaggerated, but no less important way, our necks are always adjusting to imbalances everywhere in our bodies. Since none of us have perfectly balanced bodies, to some extent we have all lost some degree of mobility and adaptability in the cervical region. Because of this loss of adaptability, you will almost always find problems with people's necks, even those who do not come to you complaining about their necks. You will find restrictions in the necks of young people and see the effects of unresolved restrictions in the severely restricted necks of older clients. The implication of these observations is significant: much of the time it will be difficult to adequately treat neck problems unless you understand and manage the imbalances and compensatory patterns in the whole body. Although this situation is especially true for the neck, it also applies to the entire body. Any time you consider manipulating a local restriction, do your best to also understand how it is related to all the other areas of compensation and strain throughout the body. If your client's body cannot adapt to or support the release of a local fixation, then either the local area will revert to its dysfunctional state or strain will be driven elsewhere—or both.

Although necks are very complicated, describing their motion is easy. With the exception of C1, all motion of the cervical spine is always Type II. When you sidebend and rotate your neck, whether you forward or back bend, and whether there are facet restrictions or not, sidebending and rotation are always coupled to the same side. This fact makes your life as a therapist a little easier. Unlike the rest of the spine, once you know how a cervical vertebra is rotated you automatically know it must be sidebent to the same side. From the previous chapters you also know that the facets on the side to which the vertebra is rotated are closed and that the facets on the opposite side are open. You could use the forward/backward bending test you learned in the last chapter to determine which facets are restricted, but if you try it you will realize rather quickly that it is not easily applied to the neck and that a different test would be useful. It turns out that there is a rather elegant motion test for determining facet restrictions, but we will save it for the next chapter. In this chapter you will learn some easy techniques that do not require knowing which facets are fixed. The rationale for this approach is based on experience and is the same as the one I explained in Chapter Two: on average, somatic practitioners tend to learn theory and technique more easily and quickly when they can get their hands to understand first.

Indirect Cervical Techniques

THE FIRST TWO TECHNIQUES WE ARE GOING TO LOOK AT ARE SIMPLE indirect techniques that do not challenge facet restrictions. They are similar to the first technique you learned for derotating lumbar and thoracic vertebrae in Chapter One. Even though these indirect techniques are not as consistently effective as the techniques that challenge the restricted facets, they can be effective on many occasions and they are fun to practice. But more importantly they can assist your learning in two very useful ways: practicing them will give you experience in feeling into and through the body, and they will also teach your hands and mind the clear difference between addressing the myofascial level and the articular level.

In order to determine whether to apply these indirect techniques the only piece of information you need to know is whether a vertebra is rotated. With your client supine, place the tips of your index fingers touching each other on one of the spinous processes of the cervical spine. Make sure that your fingers are on the same horizontal plane and that they are perpendicular to the sagittal plane. Then slowly pull your fingers laterally apart along the horizontal plane. Almost immediately you will feel your fingertips sink into the spinal groove. If the vertebra is right rotated, you will feel that your right finger is a little posterior and your left finger is a little anterior. The bump is on the right and the indentation is on the left. Test all of the cervical vertebrae in this way until you find one that is obviously rotated. And again, don't fret about the ones that are not clear. For now, just find the ones that are obviously rotated.

If you are not familiar with locating cervical vertebrae, here is a simple method for finding your way. Locate the inferior tip of the mastoid process and let your finger sink from there medially into the edge of the cervical spine. Your finger will land on the articular pillar and transverse

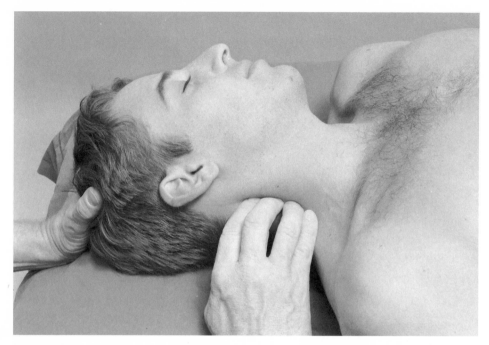

Figure 4.1

process of C2. The cervical vertebrae are spaced about a finger-width apart from each other. From C2, move down one finger-width and place your first finger on the right articular pillar of C3. Then let your other fingers fall in line under your index finger on each successive vertebrae. You now have your middle finger on C4, your ring finger on C5, and your pinky on C6 (Figure 4.1).

Figure 4.2 is a illustration of a typical cervical vertebra. The anterior and posterior tubercles in this particular vertebra constitute its transverse processes. In other cervical vertebrae, the transverse process is composed of only one prominence. Once you realize how close the articular pillars are to the tubercles, or transverse processes, you can appreciate how your fingertips, in many cases, are big enough to cover both at once. The articular pillars are also known as the articular processes. If you look at how the cervical vertebrae line up over one another, you can easily see how these articular processes function as supporting pillars.

Let's go back to your client's neck and find the most obviously rotated cervical vertebra so that you can practice the first indirect technique for

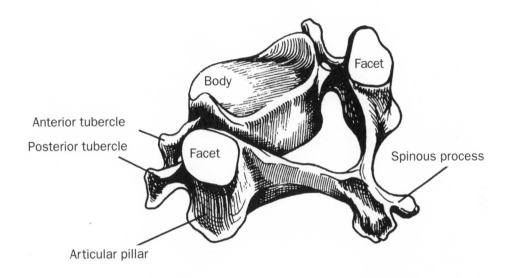

Anterior tubercle

Posterior tubercle

Facet

Body

Facet

Spinous process

Articular pillar

Figure 4.2

derotating it. Let's assume you discover that C3 is right rotated on C4. Place the tips of your thumbs on the TP's of C3 and let your forefingers sink into the spinal groove at the level of C3 (Figures 4.3 and 4.4, page 40). Gently but firmly squeeze C3 between your fingers together in the following way: press the tips of your thumbs toward each other in a medial direction as you squeeze your forefingers into the spinal groove in an anterior and slightly superior direction. Wait and you will feel the marvelous response of your client's body to your touch as it begins to correct itself. You will probably first feel C3 move further into right rotation and right sidebending and then change direction and possibly move toward left rotation and left sidebending, perhaps moving in unpredictable and surprising ways before it settles and releases. Don't try to anticipate its motion, just follow the dance. When it releases you will feel the associated tissues soften and the neck organize itself along the sagittal plane. If the technique was successful your client will report that his pain is either gone or lessened and you will notice that C3 is no longer right rotated. Practice this technique for a while until you try the next one.

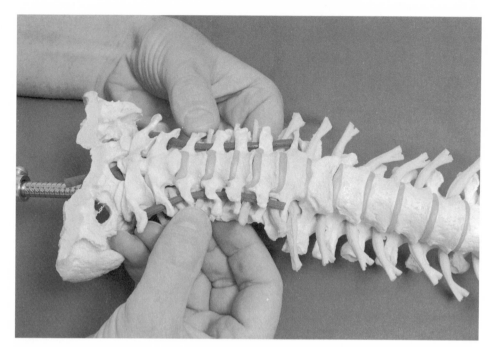

Figure 4.3

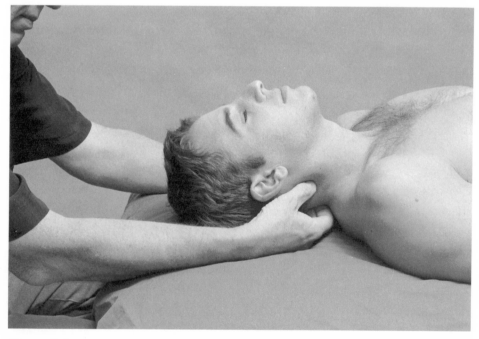

Figure 4.4

The second indirect technique is not only simple, but rather elegant. It was created by my friend and colleague, Jan Sultan, who jokingly and appropriately calls it "Dial-a-Neck." You may find this technique a little more effective than the previous one because it involves larger movements of the head and neck which may, in turn, have more of an effect on the facet restrictions.

Grasp the TP's of C3 between the thumb and middle finger of your right hand (Figures 4.5, 4.6, and 4.7). With your left hand grasp the top of your client's head and rotate it to the right so that its rotation, according to your best guess, matches the rotation of C3. Now wait for a moment and you will experience a remarkable development—C3 and your client's head will both begin to move further into right rotation. Just follow this motion until the head and neck rotate no further and wait. In a few seconds you may feel a slight pulsation under your fingers (it doesn't really matter whether you feel this pulsation or not; but since many therapists do feel it, it is worth mentioning). Continue to wait for a few more moments and you will feel an impulse in your client's neck and head to come out

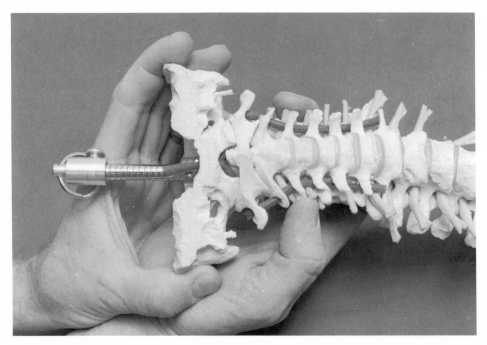

Figure 4.5

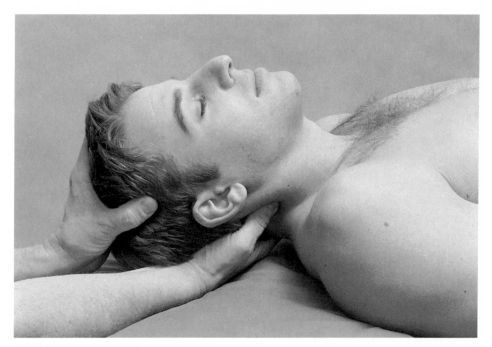

Figure 4.6

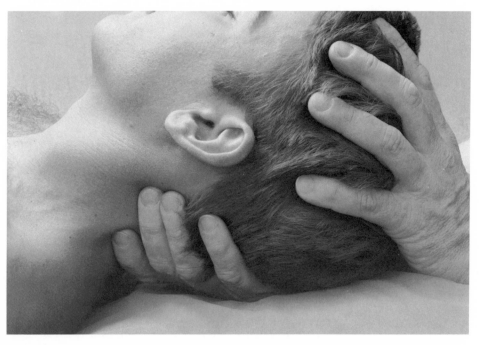

Figure 4.7

of its extreme rotation. Again, just follow the directions in which the head and neck want to move. They may rotate to the left and then back to the right as they sidebend, forward and backward bend, this way and that. Don't impose your notions of what is possible or what you think they should do, just follow the dance. Eventually, the head and neck will cease all sidebending and rotating, and settle in a straight line. Wait for the tissues to soften under your fingers and for the orthotropic effect as the neck lengthens and organizes itself along the sagittal axis. Palpate C3 and see if it derotated. If the technique was successful, C3 will no longer be rotated, the tissues will feel more relaxed, and your client will report that his pain is lessened or completely gone.

You may have noticed that my favorite expression for how to respond to the body as it finds normal is "Just follow the dance." The refined aesthetic sensibilities of some Italian students that I once taught in Rome led them to coin the phrase, "The Dance of the Tissues" to describe this astonishing ability of the body to find its way back home when given permission. With a little practice and patience everyone can learn to perceive this dance. All it requires is that you let go of your tendency to anticipate and comment on the process that is unfolding under your hands and let what is happening unfold in its own way. Resist the temptation to step out of the flow of lived-experience and reflect on what is happening.

Reflectively thinking about experience certainly has a place in life, but not when you are applying these techniques. Athletes sometimes refer to this pre-reflective way of being and doing as the "Zone." If a basketball player were to think to himself as he was about to score the winning point in the last seconds of the game, "Oh, this is great I am about to score two big ones," he probably wouldn't. If, during an inspired performance, a great concert musician were to continually comment to herself, "I am playing this beautifully, Mozart would be so impressed!" her inspiration would soon become a fleeting memory. In the same way, if you reflect on the process or comment to yourself in elation, skepticism, or self-doubt, you will just as surely lose your ability to follow the dance of the tissues.

All too often when therapists first attempt to follow the dance of the tissues they adopt all sorts of silent, self-defeating monologues and attitudes that instantly hinder their ability to feel the obvious. Since they are often not prepared for the experience of the body moving under its own

43

direction independently of their or the client's conscious control, they doubt what they are feeling. Sometimes their skepticism gets in their way and they think, "Oh, this can't be happening!" and suddenly what they were feeling disappears under their hands. At other times their own astonishment brings the dance to a complete standstill. Before they even touch the body, some therapists assume that they are not sensitive enough to feel such movements and just as surely as they let their feelings of inadequacy take over, they lose their innate ability to follow the dance of the tissues. However, you can learn to put all such notions aside and just let yourself *feel* what the body wants to do.

The most common mistake that beginning followers of the dance make is to anticipate what the body wants to do as it transitions from one position to another. At first they find themselves following the dance quite well as the body continues to rotate and sidebend in one direction. But at the very moment the body stops moving in the direction they are following and begins to shift in another direction, they immediately wonder what is happening, although more than likely they will not even form a complete thought about it. Either the momentary cessation of movement in a clear direction or a slow but obvious change of direction compels them to instinctively wonder about what is going on. It is much like what happens when you see movement from the corner of your eye—you instinctively and inquisitively turn to see what the movement is. Although no words may be spoken, your orientation and comportment say "What's that?"

It doesn't really matter what therapists say or don't say to themselves when the body changes directions during treatment. What matters is that they step out of the flow of lived-experience and lose track of the dance. If you are not pre-reflectively there to follow the body's lead, you are no longer able to recognize its pattern of strain—there is no longer anything for you to follow and so you stop moving. Since it takes two to tango, the body also stops moving. If this happens to you during the transitions, all that you need to do is simply stop thinking about what you are feeling. Let go of your surprise, puzzlement, or wordless "What's that?" and just feel again how the body slow dances toward its own correction.

Learning to work this way is an exercise in learning how not to think, how not to worry, and how to be happy with what is. The more you learn to live in this place of no-thinking, the happier you will become. Explore this open way of not reflectively thinking about what is occurring, because it is a gateway into the healer's way of being that I briefly mentioned in the introduction. Explore this spacious way of being when you are not working with clients and you can transform your life. Explore it while working with your clients and their bodies will reveal more and more of what they need from you. In time you will be less and less concerned about imposing your will and presuppositions on your clients, or the world, and things will unfold with an impeccable clarity.

Like most indirect techniques of this nature Dial-a-Neck will sometimes produce wonderful and astounding results and at other times it will seem like a waste of effort. Now you know why—it's because these techniques do not directly challenge joint fixations. Since we are approaching all joint fixations in this book from the soft-tissue perspective, we need a way to challenge the joint fixation without resorting to high-velocity, low-amplitude thrusting techniques, and that is what the next technique will accomplish.

A Joint Challenging Technique

THIS JOINT-CHALLENGING TECHNIQUE IS VERY LIKE THE SHOTGUN technique you learned in Chapter Two to release facet restrictions in the thoracic and lumbar sections of the spine. Although there are a number of small differences, let me describe the technique simply, without mentioning these differences so you know you are in familiar territory. It works just as you might expect: you locate the rotated vertebra and assume that it is fixed closed on the side to which it is rotated and fixed open on the opposite side, put pressure on the fixed-closed facets in forward bending and wait for the release, and put pressure on the fixed-open facets in backward bending and wait for the release.

You will be happy to learn that this shotgun technique does not waste as much time when applied to the cervical spine. In the thoracic or lumbar spines, the facets are either fixed open or fixed closed. So every time you apply this shotgun approach to a lumbar or thoracic vertebra, you are always addressing one side too many. But the cervical spine is different. Very often you will find that the facets on both sides are fixed. It is very common to find a cervical vertebra that is bilaterally restricted with facets that are fixed closed on one side and fixed open on the other side. Your efficiency, therefore, goes up somewhat when you use this technique for the neck.

There are some important differences between the vertebra of the neck and the rest of the spine that you need to understand. One of these differences is reason for caution. There are two vertebral arteries that run along and inside the cervical vertebrae and irritating or cutting them off, especially in older clients, can be very dangerous. The vertebral arteries are especially at risk at C6, C7, and at the occiptioatlantal junction. Even if your arteries are normal, when you rotate your neck they can narrow as much as 90% on the side opposite the rotation. Forward bending and sidebending the neck will not put these arteries at risk, but back bending will greatly exaggerate what happens in rotation. Back bending a client's neck while applying a high-velocity, low-amplitude thrusting technique, for example, is a very dangerous approach. Be careful. When you are attempting to release open fixed cervical facets, even using the soft-tissue techniques taught in this book, you must modify them and not put your clients's neck very far into extension.

If you put your client into back bending and rotation by mistake and she complains of dizziness or you notice that her eyes begin to move involuntarily in a rhythmic back and forth pattern (known as nystagmus) take her out of extension immediately and suggest that she see her doctor. If you have any doubts about the integrity of a client's vertebral arteries, there is a simple test you can apply. Put your client in a sitting position with her spine comfortably straight. Ask her to back bend her head and then turn her head to the right and to the left. Watch for the appearance of nystagmus or dizziness.

Since the neck is capable of more motion than the rest of the spine, you can introduce sidebending and rotation as a way to further challenge facet restrictions. In fact, you should use sidebending and rotation in place of introducing significant extension as you manipulate open fixed facets. In the case of closed-fixed facets, you can apply extreme forward bending without worry when you apply sidebending and rotation.

Notice also how the facets are arranged in the cervical spine. Not only are they are almost parallel to the transverse plane, the facets are accessible to your fingers in three places: in the spinal groove, at the lateral edges where the articular pillars and transverse processes are, and just slightly anterior and medial to the articular pillars and transverse processes. Having a number of places where the facets are accessible to your fingers makes the application of this technique just a little bit easier, because you can adjust the application of pressure to allow for how the body is best able to release.

So let's take a more careful look at this technique. For the purposes of illustration, assume again that C3 is right rotated on C4. Either the right facets are fixed closed or the left facets are fixed open—or both sides are fixed. Since C3 is right rotated, you know that it also must be right sidebent. If it is right sidebent, it will be restricted in left sidebending and rotation, which means that it can easily sidebend and rotate right, but cannot sidebend and rotate left. You need to know the direction in which C3 cannot sidebend and rotate in order to challenge the facets.

Release the right facets first. Cradle the back of your client's head in your left hand and lift it off the table. Lean your elbow on the table so that you can comfortably support your client's head. Then left sidebend and left rotate your client's head and neck as far as they will comfortably go. Forward bending and sidebending both challenge the presumed fixed-closed right facets. Then put your index or middle finger on the presumed fixed closed facets in the right spinal groove or on the articular pillars, as shown in Figure 4.8, page 48. As you keep your client's head in its left-sidebent position, let your finger sink into the spinal groove and wait. When the facets release, you will notice the usual indicators: softening of the tissue and a sense of the neck lengthening along the sagittal plane. But you will also feel something else. Remember that C3 is not able to sidebend and rotate left because of the presumed right-fixed facets. When the facets release, you will also feel your client's head and neck left sidebend and rotate just a little further. If these are the only facets restricted in the neck, then the left sidebending and rotation will be very obvious.

Now let's release the presumed fixed-open facets on the left. Again, cradle the back of your client's head in your right hand, lift it up, and rest your elbow on the table. Put your left index or middle finger on the fixed open facets by placing your left finger in the left spinal groove or between the articular pillars as shown in Figures 4.9 and 4.10, page 49. To make things easier for yourself, allow your client's head to rest on the webbing

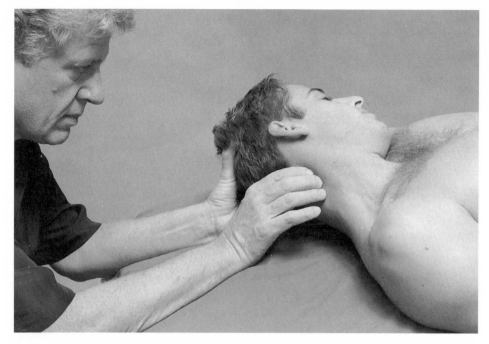

Figure 4.8

between the thumb and forefinger of your left hand. Push ever so slightly in an anterior direction to give just the suggestion of back bending. With your right hand, sidebend and rotate your client's head and neck to the left as far as they will comfortably go and wait. When the facets release, you will feel the tissues soften, the sense of lengthening along the sagittal plane, and your client's head and neck turning further into left sidebending and rotation.

It is a good idea to experiment with and modify this technique a bit. Try different placements of your left index finger. See how the technique works for you when you put your index finger in the spinal groove, between the TP's of C3 and C4, or just slightly in front of and between the TP's of C3 and C4 as you sidebend and rotate your client's head and neck to the left. Also, you don't have to wait passively for the facets to release. Experiment with gently twisting and jiggling your client's head in the direction of left sidebending as you apply pressure either on the open or closed facets. You can also very effectively combine the direct and indirect approaches. By twisting and then jiggling your client's head and neck in the

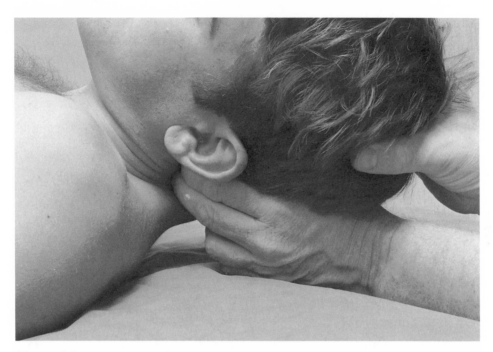

Figure 4.9

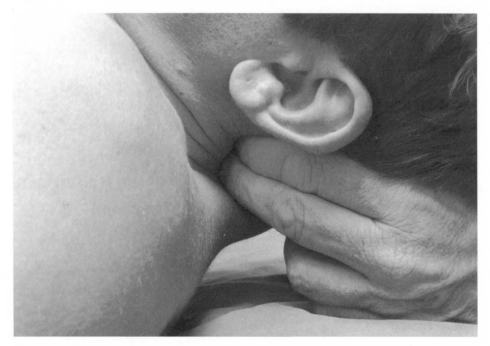

Figure 4.10

direction it cannot sidebend and rotate, you are challenging the facet restriction by performing a direct technique. But if you then wait for your client's body to respond to your direct challenge and follow the dance of the tissues you are approaching the fixation indirectly. Try jiggling and rotating while waiting for the dance, and then more jiggling and rotating and again waiting for the dance, and so on until you secure a satisfactory release. Don't be surprised if you have to perform the technique a couple of times to completely release the fixation.

This joint-challenging technique can also be used with a new motion test for determining which facets are fixed and how they are fixed. That you will learn in the next chapter. The test will allow you to be more efficient in your approach and provide an important indicator of facet fixation. Remember that fixation is more important than position. Checking for rotation before and after the application of a technique is not a perfectly reliable indicator of dysfunction or its release. A vertebra may appear to have derotated and yet not have been completely released from its facet restriction. You should also realize that a vertebra can appear to be slightly rotated and not actually have any facet restrictions. The motion testing that you are about to learn will give you a very clear way to know, without relying on palpating rotation, whether you have discovered cervical facet restrictions and whether you were successful in releasing them.

5

Motion Testing the Cervical Spine

T HE MOTION TEST DEVELOPED BY OSTEOPATHS FOR DETERMINING facet restrictions in the cervical spine is called the Translation Test. Translation in this context refers to motion induced along a straight or curved plane. The test is simple and quite elegant: you forward bend and backward bend your client's head and neck and then push each vertebra from right to left and from left to right along a horizontal plane. If you find that the vertebra moves from right to left but not from left to right, you have discovered a facet restriction.

When you hold your client's neck in forward bending while you translate the vertebra, you are testing to see if the facets can open. If there are no facet restrictions, the facets will open in forward bending and you will be able to translate the vertebra from left to right and right to left. However, if you find that you can translate from right to left, but not from left to right in forward bending, you have discovered fixed closed facets that will not permit translatory motion. Likewise, when you put your client's neck in a back bending position and translate, you are testing for whether the facets can close. If you find that you cannot translate from right to left with your client's neck in backward bending, then you have discovered fixed open facets that will not permit translatory motion.

The absence of translatory motion indicates the location of the facet restriction. In the forward bending position, loss of motion indicates fixed-closed facets and in the backward bending position, loss of motion indicates fixed-open facets. In the forward bending position the facet restriction is on the side opposite the motion restriction and in the backward bending position the facet restriction is on the same side as the motion restriction. This may sound odd, or even paradoxical at first, but it makes perfectly good sense once you understand the logic of the test and the Type II biomechanics of C2–C7.

Don't concern yourself with the logic of the test just yet or with how to determine on which side the facet restriction is. We will get to these important aspects of the test soon enough. Before we do, there is an important distinction to keep in mind. Not understanding or hearing this simple distinction at the outset has been enough to drive some rather intelligent and normal therapists around the bend. The distinction is between a *facet restriction* and a *motion restriction.*

A facet restriction is the cause of the motion restriction. If you cannot translate a cervical vertebra in one direction, the cause of this lack of motion is a facet restriction. After you apply this test you then use the discovery of the motion restriction to deduce where the facet restriction is. Unlike what you learned in the forward and backward bending tests for the thoracic and lumbar spines, you will be deducing facet restrictions from motion restrictions in the cervical spine, not from the how the vertebra appears to derotate. Remember this distinction and that you are taking your reference point from motion restriction, not from rotation.

In order to understand what translation is and how it works, practice it with your client's head lying comfortably on the treatment table, making sure that his neck is relatively straight. Admittedly, this position is not very useful for getting the information you need for determining facet restrictions. You must use translation in the forward and back bending positions to get that information. However, we are practicing translation this way first so that you can understand how it works without the added effort of maintaining your client's head and neck in forward and backward bending.

Let's start by translating C3 with your client's head and neck lying comfortably straight on the table. Find C3 and place your index and middle fingers on each TP. Use your palms and thenar eminences to stabilize and hold the upper part of the cervical spine and the head. Introduce translation by moving your fingers and hands (as a whole, as if their were no

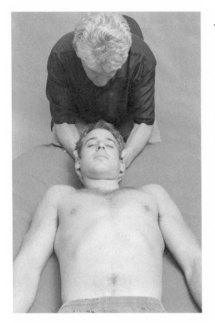

Figure 5.1

joints in your hands) from left to right and from right to left along the horizontal plane (Figure 5.1). Be certain that you are introducing motion only along the horizontal plane — be very careful not to actually sidebend your client's neck. The neck and C3 will automatically sidebend as a result of moving it along the horizontal. If you inadvertently sidebend your client while you are attempting to translate C3, you will not get a clear reading. Feel what happens under your fingers. Does C3 move better left to right or right to left? If you are not sure check C2 through C7 until you find a vertebra that clearly does not move as easily in one direction as it does the other. Don't worry yet about how to interpret your findings. You may actually find some vertebrae that don't translate at all. Ignore these cases until you find a vertebra that obviously translates one way and not the other. Just make sure you are translating correctly and not inadvertently introducing sidebending into your motion. Do you notice how translation alone is sufficient to create sidebending?

Once you are comfortable with translating C2–C7, try translating C3 in the forward bending position. Prop your elbows on the table. Cradle and stabilize your client's head and cervical vertebrae above C3 with your palms and thenar eminences and lift the head off the table (Figure 5.2, page 54). It is very important that you prop up your elbows so that you are not exerting a lot of unnecessary effort trying to hold your client's head still. Many clients have a difficult time relinquishing control of their necks to your hands, so the more stable and secure they feel in your hands, the more they can give up control. If you cannot comfortably manage this position for yourself, you might try using a face cradle for your table that will allow your client's head to rest easily on it in the forward and backward bending positions (Figure 5.3).

In any case, put your client's neck in flexion by lifting it off the table.

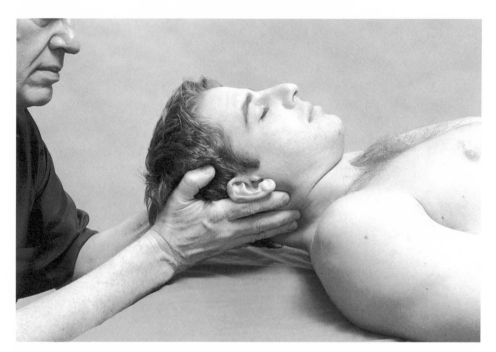

Figure 5.2

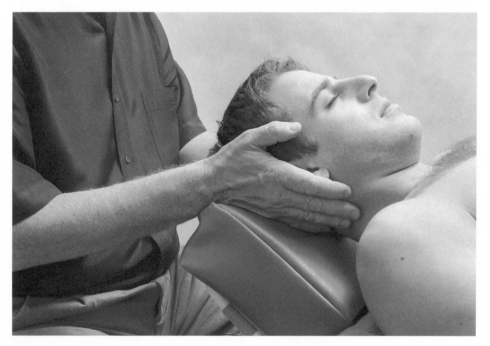

Figure 5.3

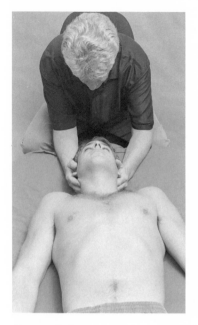

Figure 5.4

Stabilize the head and C1–C2 with your palms and thenar eminences, and then translate C3 along the horizontal plane from right to left and then from left to right. Does it translate better one way than another? If so, you have discovered a motion restriction that will allow you to deduce the side on which the facets are fixed closed. If C3 translates from right to left, but not from left to right, the motion restriction is on the left. Don't concern yourself right now with how to deduce the side with the fixed-closed facets from the discovery of motion restriction, just feel the restriction. If C3 translates both ways, go looking for a vertebra that doesn't.

Now try translating in the backward bending position. To achieve an easy extension of the neck, simply slide the lateral edge of your forefinger under the neck and gently push it in an anterior direction while you simultaneously and gently push your client's head in an inferior position. Stabilize the head and C1–C2 with your palms and thenar eminences, and translate C3 first one way and then the other (Figure 5.4). If you find that C3 translates one way better than another, you have discovered a motion restriction that will allow you to deduce the side on which the facets are fixed open. If C3 translates from left to right, but not from right to left, the motion restriction is on the right. Again, don't concern yourself at this point with learning which side is fixed open, just learn to feel for the motion restriction. If you don't find a motion restriction at C3 on C4, then test other cervical vertebrae until you find a motion restriction.

Practice translation on all the cervical vertebrae with the exception of C1: in forward and backward bending until you are fairly confident that you can locate each individual vertebra and feel its free or restricted motion. After practicing on a number of different clients, you will be amazed at the profound differences between necks. Some necks seem to be very flexible, with supple soft tissues, and yet still show facet restrictions. Other necks seem to be tight and rigid at every level. Of course, you will find those necks that seem at first as though they should be fixated at every level, but are relatively free of facet restrictions. What experience teaches you is that everyone is different and that the feeling of a restriction in one person may be unrestricted motion for another. Ultimately, no matter what part of the body you are evaluating, you must learn to feel what constitutes a restriction for each individual person.

Now that you have some familiarity with translation, let's look a little more closely at the motion test and the information you can glean from it. Translation automatically introduces sidebending and rotation to the same side. Since sidebending and rotation are always coupled to the same side in the neck (with the exception of C1), if you know which direction a vertebra cannot sidebend, you also know the way it cannot rotate. Regardless of whether you translate your client's neck in forward or backward bending, if C3 can translate from the right to the left, but not from the left to the right, you immediately know that the vertebra is right sidebent and right rotated, with fixed facets somewhere that are preventing left sidebending and left rotation.

Figuring out which facets are restricted is quite simple. Suppose in forward bending you can translate C3 from right to left, but not from left to right. The discovery of a motion restriction on the left means that C3 is right sidebent and right rotated on C4 and that C3 cannot left sidebend and left rotate. Since you are testing in forward bending, you also know that you have discovered fixed closed facets. So since C3 has facets that are fixed closed and C3 is right sidebent and right rotated, then you know the fixed closed facets must be on the right.

Suppose you test another client's neck in back bending and you find the same motion restriction. In back bending you discover a motion restriction on the left: C3 translates easily from right to left but, not from left to right. This discovery tells you that C3 is right sidebent and right rotated and cannot left sidebend and left rotate. Since you are testing in back bending, you know that you have discovered fixed open facets. Since C3 is right sidebent and right rotated on C4 and the facets are fixed open, you know that the fixed open facets must be on the left.

Two simple rules immediately emerge from this exercise: 1) when you translate in forward bending and meet a motion restriction, the facets are fixed closed on the side opposite to the motion restriction, and 2) when you translate in back bending and meet a motion restriction, the facets are fixed open on the same side as the motion restriction.

Don't let your memory of the forward and backward bending tests for the thoracic and lumbar spines confuse your understanding of the translation test. Remember that for the cervical spine you are deducing where the facet restriction is from determining where the motion restriction is. You are not deducing the location of the facet restriction from how the vertebra appears to derotate, as you did in the thoracic and lumbar spines. The reference point you are using to deduce the facet restriction in the cervical spine, is motion restriction, not rotation. For the thoracic and lumbar spines, you deduce that the fixed-closed facets are on the same side as the rotation and that the fixed-open facets are on the opposite side of the rotation. In the cervical spine, you deduce that the fixed-closed facets are on the side opposite to the motion restriction and that the fixed open facets are on the same side as the motion restriction. With cervical translation, the reference point—the side to which the facet fixation is either opposite or the same—is reversed in relation to the forward and backward bending test for the thoracic and lumbar spines.

Why does it work this way? Let's stick with the same example. If there are no fixed-closed facets, then when you forward bend your client's neck all the facets will open and when you translate you will not meet any motion restriction. When you translate in forward bending and meet a motion restriction, the cause is fixed closed facets. In our example translation tells you that C3 is right sidebent and right rotated on C4 and that the right facets are fixed closed. When you translate right to left the left facets must be free to open to allow that motion to occur. Since the left facets are indeed free to open, you are able to translate right to left. But when you try to translate left to right the situation changes. Translating left to right can only happen if the right facets can open. But since they are fixed closed, they cannot open and will not permit left-to-right translation. You feel the motion restriction on the left, because the right facets will not open, and are fixed closed. You do not feel the motion restriction on the right because the left facets are able to open as you translate right to left.

When you back bend your client's neck, if there are no fixed-open facets, all the cervical facets will close and you will not meet any motion restrictions when you translate. If you meet a motion restriction while translating in back bending, the cause is fixed open facets. Translation tells you that C3 is right sidebent and right rotated on C4 and that the left facets are fixed open. In back bending, when you translate from right to left, the right facets must be capable of closing for that motion to occur. Since the right facets are free and able to close, you can easily translate from right to left. In order for you to be able to translate C3 from left to right, the left facets must be capable of closing. But since they are fixed open, they cannot close, and hence you cannot translate C3 from left to right. You feel the motion restriction on the left, because the left facets will not close, because they are fixed open. You do not feel the motion restriction on the right, because the right facets are able to close to permit translation from right to left.

After translating the necks of a number of people, you may notice a rather common occurrence, in which you meet a motion restriction on the same side in both forward and backward bending. For example, suppose you find that you can translate C4 from left to right but not from right to left in both forward and backward bending. When you discover a case like this where the motion restriction is on the right in both forward and backward bending, it means that the facets on both sides are fixed. The left facets are fixed closed and the right facets are fixed open. If you detect a motion restriction on the left in both forward and back bending, it means that the right facets are fixed closed and the left facets are fixed open.

You will also encounter necks that exhibit motion restriction on both sides in both forward and backward bending. Bilateral motion restriction can be the result of arthritis or something simple, like rigid tight muscles and fasciae. In the latter case, you must release these myofascial restrictions first.

When you are first learning how to motion test the neck for facet restrictions, do not confuse yourself by trying to elucidate the logic of the test. Just learn to feel for motion restrictions and use the simple rules provided to deduce the facet restriction. Unlike the forward and backward bending tests for the thoracics and lumbars, cervical translation involves not only sidebending, rotation, forward bending, and backward bending, but also left and right translation. Trying to understand the results of the test while attempting to remember all these conditions can become very complicated. So here are the simple rules for C2–C7:

If translation reveals a motion restriction in *backward* bending, then the facets are *fixed open* on the *same side* as the motion restriction.

If translation reveals a motion restriction in *forward* bending, then the facets are *fixed closed* on the *side opposite* to the motion restriction.

As with the other rules provided, you can reformulate these any way that suits your understanding. If you memorize these rules or keep a copy where you can see them, you will save yourself a lot of grief as you work with your clients. If you are like most therapists, you do not want to try to think your way through the logic of these tests while you are applying them—you just want to apply the tests so that you can quickly determine which facets are fixed.

If you have been practicing the shotgun techniques from Chapter 3 that challenge cervical facet restrictions, then you already know how to release them. The translation test gives you the added ability to locate more precisely where and how the facet is restricted. The translation test has another great advantage. As previously noted, if your only way of knowing whether a cervical facet restriction has been released is the appearance of derotation, then you do not have a fully reliable indicator. Translation gives you a far more accurate way to determine whether the facet has been released than checking for derotation.

As you practice these techniques, allow yourself the freedom to let the client's body tell you how it wants to release itself. When you rotate and sidebend the head and neck to challenge a facet restriction, sometimes the body wants to rotate and sidebend to the opposite side before it releases. Be prepared to follow the dance of the tissues, even if it means following the body into seemingly odd positions. Learn to easily shift from direct to indirect techniques and back again as the body demands. When you begin with challenging a facet restriction, wait to see how the body responds to your invitation. The head and neck may want to rotate and sidebend to the side opposite to how you are holding them. They may want to go into flexion and then extension as they sidebend and rotate this way and that until they finally release. Or the facets may simply go directly into a release in the direction you are encouraging it to go.

Always check the results of your work. After you have applied a tech-nique, translate the cervical vertebra again to make sure you released the facet restriction completely. Don't be surprised if you have to apply the technique a few times before the facets release to your satisfaction. Unlike the techniques you learned for releasing the rest of the spine, the cervi-cal vertebrae sometimes require a few applications of the technique until the facets release.

In the next chapter you will learn how to release atlas-on-axis restric-tions and occiput-on-atlas restrictions.

6

The Atlas and Occiput

T O COMPLETE YOUR UNDERSTANDING OF THE NECK YOU NEED TO KNOW how to release atlas on axis (AA) restrictions and occiput on atlas (OA) restrictions. The techniques are similar to what you have already learned and are very easy to apply.

Ninety percent of normal atlas motion on the axis is rotation. There is some sidebending, but from a clinical standpoint it is not important enough to worry about. When the atlas gets in trouble, it is due to restricted rotation. You can determine whether C1 is rotated on C2 by palpating for whether one TP is anterior and the other is posterior, but in many necks C1 rotation is sometimes difficult to feel. Besides, sometimes the atlas can be slightly rotated and show no restricted facets. In general, the most reliable way to determine dysfunction is by using a simple motion test.

Begin with your client in a supine position on your treatment table. Grasp his head with both hands and flex the cervical spine so that the head is lifted up about 45 degrees. Positioning the cervical spine in this way locks C2–C7 and forces the atlas to rotate with the occiput. Maintain the cervical spine in this position and rotate your client's head to the left and then to the right (Figures 6.1 and 6.2, page 62). If C1 is not restricted on C2, then you will be able to easily and obviously rotate his head freely to each side. If the atlas rotation is restricted, you will be able to rotate his head easily in one direction, but not as far in the other. So if his head rotates to the right and not as well to the left, C1 is right rotated and

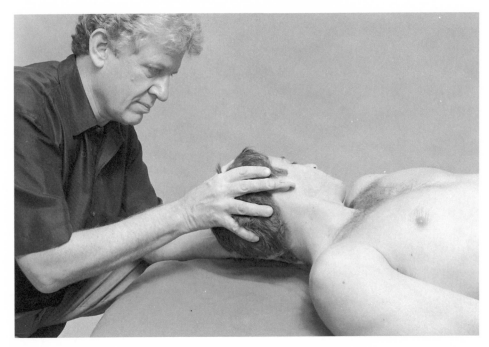

Figure 6.1

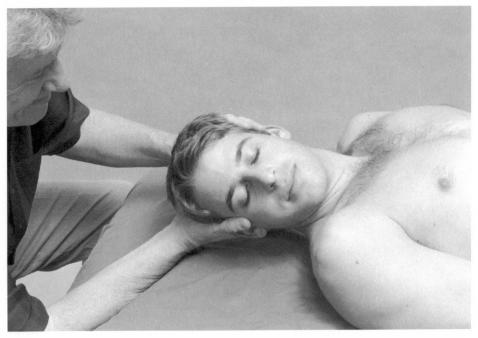

Figure 6.2

restricted in left rotation. If his head rotates better to the left than the right, then the atlas is left rotated and restricted in right rotation.

Releasing the atlas is easy: keep your client's head in 45 degrees flexion and rotate it in the direction it is restricted. If the test shows you that the atlas is left rotated, turn his head to the right as far as it can comfortably go. Place your right index and/or middle fingers on the posterior arch of the atlas close to the posterior surface of the right transverse process (Figure 6.3, page 64) and let the full weight of his head rest on your fingers (Figure 6.4). Make sure you do not place your fingers on the tip of the right transverse process of the atlas. Not only will this technique not work with this finger placement, it will also create unnecessary pain for your client. Just let his weight rest on your fingers while you wait for the release. You will feel all the familiar indications of release as his head an atlas begin to slowly rotate more and more to the right. You can either wait for the tissues to release or encourage the release by gently turning and/or jiggling his head to the right. Retest to make sure you have completely released the rotation restriction. It may take more than one application of this technique to completely release the atlas.

Restrictions of the occiput on the atlas are very common and if not released these restrictions will come back to haunt you. The most sterling and profound releases of the C1–C7 often will not relieve your client's pain if you do not address the influence of the occiput. Sometimes an OA restriction is enough to reestablish an AA restriction even after the AA restriction has been released. And over time those restrictions can be responsible for other restrictions showing up throughout your client's spine.

Whether normal or abnormal, in both forward or backward bending, all motion of the occiput on the atlas is Type I. There are no discs between the occiput and the atlas, and the joints do not open and close in forward and backward bending the way they do in the rest of the spine. Rather the convex condyles of the occiput glide posteriorly on the superior concave facets of the atlas when you forward bend and glide anteriorly on the atlas when you backward bend. When you sidebend to the right, for example, the right condyle will slide inferiorly on a facet of the atlas and the left condyle will slide superiorly. If you find an OA restriction, you can say that the occiput is fixed in extension (or backward bending) or in flexion (or

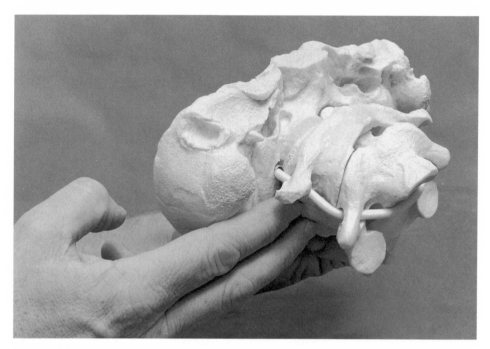

Figure 6.3

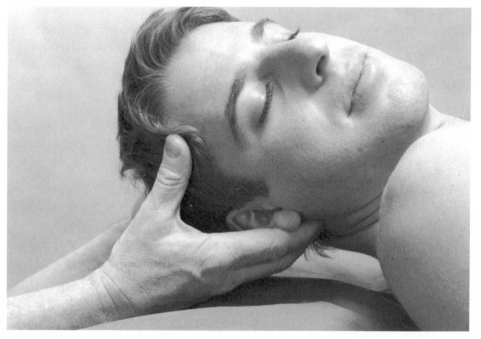

Figure 6.4

forward bending). Since the condyles do not open and close in forward and backward bending, you cannot say that they are fixed closed or fixed open.

You can reliably test for restrictions of the occiput on the atlas by using the lateral translation test. If you meet a restriction while translating in forward bending, it means that the occipital condyle cannot glide posteriorly because it is fixed anteriorly, in extension, or back bending. If you meet a motion restriction while translating in backward bending it means that the occipital condyle cannot glide anteriorly because it is fixed posteriorly, in flexion, or forward bending.

You can easily and quickly release OA restrictions by using a technique that is almost the same as the one you learned for releasing the atlas. The only difference between the two techniques is where you place your fingers.

To locate the restriction, translate your client's head from right to left and from left to right in both flexion and extension. Suppose you find that you can translate your client's occiput from left to right but not from right to left in forward bending. Since translation introduces sidebending and you are testing in forward bending, finding a motion restriction on the right means that his occiput is left sidebent and right rotated and fixed in extension, or backward bending. To release this back-bending restriction, keep his head and neck in the forward-bending position to challenge the facet restriction. Sidebend and rotate him in the direction he cannot sidebend, which in this case is to the right. Place your right index and middle fingers on the base of the occiput near the right occipital condlye and let the full weight of his head rest on your fingers (Figure 6.5, page 66). Again, either just wait for the release or encourage the release by gently turning, sidebending and/or jiggling his head to the right. You will feel the tissues soften while his head slowly sidebends and turns right. Retest to make sure you released the restriction completely.

The test and technique are basically the same in the backward bending position. Backward bend your client's head and neck and translate the occiput both ways. If his head translates easily from right to left but not from left to right, then you know that the occiput is right sidebent, left rotated, and fixed in flexion or forward bending. To release this forward-bending restriction, keep his head in a back bending position and sidebend and turn it to the left while resting the base of the occiput—

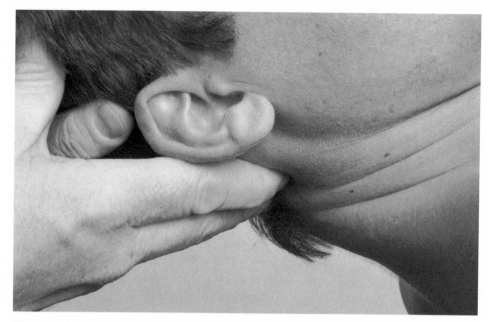

Figure 6.5

near the left occipital condyle—on your left index and middle fingers. Again, just wait for the release or encourage the release by gently turning and/or jiggling the head more to the left. You will feel the tissues soften as his head sidebends and turns left. Be sure to retest your results and don't be surprised if it takes more than one application to adequately release OA restrictions.

Describing the biomechanics of OA restrictions can be complicated, but testing for and releasing them, as you have discovered, is fairly straight-forward. If translation reveals a motion restriction in forward or backward bending, you sidebend and turn the head in the direction it won't trans-late, which is the direction in which it cannot sidebend. Keep the head in either forward or backward bending, depending on which position you find the motion restriction, and apply pressure accordingly—that's all there is to it.

You may be tempted to formulate a rule for yourself like the following: when you translate the occiput on the atlas in forward and backward bend-ing the side on which you meet the motion restriction is the side on which the facet restriction is found. The technique actually works as if this rule were correct, but it's not. When you meet a motion restriction in forward bending the facet restriction is on the side opposite the motion restriction. In backward bending the facet restriction is on the same side as the motion restriction. In backward bending it makes good clinical sense to both turn your client's head in the direction of the motion restriction and apply your pressure to the side of the motion restriction. But in forward bending, since the facet restriction is on the side opposite the motion restriction, although it makes good sense to turn your client's head in the direction of the motion restriction, it doesn't seem sensible to apply your pressure to the side of the motion restriction. You would think it would be more effective to apply your pressure to the side opposite the motion restriction. Interestingly, the technique works quite well in forward bending, but I don't know exactly why it does. I could speculate about why and how it works, but I am not sure that would further your technical skills. Instead let's look at why the rule is not correct and try to come up with a rule that reflects the specifics of what is actually going on and that will allow you to be more specific in how you apply the technique.

When you back bend and translate the occiput on the atlas, you are testing for whether the occipital condyles can glide anteriorly. If you find a motion restriction it means that one of condyles is fixed posteriorly. When you forward bend and translate the occiput, you are trying to determine whether the condyles can glide posteriorly. Finding a motion restriction indicates that one of the condyles is fixed anteriorly. To formulate the correct rule we need to know how to deduce the fixed condyle from a motion restriction.

Suppose you translate your client's occiput in back bending and discover that it can translate from left to right, but not from right to left. Since you know that the occiput always sidebends and rotates to opposite sides, the discovery of this motion restriction tells you that the occiput is left sidebent and right rotated. In back bending, since translation tests for the ability of the condyles to glide anteriorly, if you meet a motion restriction you also know that one of the condyles is fixed in flexion or forward bending. If it is fixed in flexion or forward bending, then it is fixed posteriorly. You now have all the information you need to figure out the side on which the condyle is fixed. If the occiput is right rotated, then the right side of the occiput is posterior and the left side is anterior. If it is fixed posteriorly and right rotated, the posterior fixation must be on the right.

Why does it work this way? In back bending, translation of the occiput requires that the occipital condyles glide anteriorly. When you meet a motion restriction translating right to left it means that the right condyle is fixed posteriorly and will not permit anterior glide. You can translate the other way, from left to right, because the left condyle is not fixed and will permit anterior glide. Since the right condyle is fixed posteriorly, left sidebent, and right rotated, when you translate from left to right, the occiput sidebends left and rotates right. As a result, the left occipital condyle glides anteriorly and sidebends left, while the right side of the occiput slides posteriorly, in the direction it is already rotated and posteriorly fixed. So when you translate the occiput in back bending, you will feel the motion restriction on the same side as the facet restriction.

Now suppose you translate your client's occiput in forward bending and meet a motion restriction going from right to left, but not from left to right. The facet restriction is on the left, the side opposite to the motion restriction. But how do you get to this conclusion? Finding the motion restriction on the right tells you that the occiput is left sidebent, right rotated, and that one of the condyles is fixed anteriorly because it is unable to glide posteriorly. Once you know that the occiput is right rotated and one condyle is fixed anteriorly, you know that the anteriorly fixed condyle has to be on the left. If the occiput is right rotated, it is posterior on the right and anterior on the left. Since translation revealed that a condyle is fixed anteriorly, you know that the fixation must be on the left.

You can probably figure out yourself why it works this way in forward bending, but let's go through the logic of it. In order for the occiput to translate both ways, the condyles must be capable of gliding anteriorly. In the above example, the motion restriction is on the right. The occiput can translate from left to right because it is capable of sidebending left while the left condyle glides anteriorly. As the left condyle glides anteriorly the occiput rotates right. Since the right condyle is already right rotated and posterior, it can glide in that direction. But in order for you to translate the occiput from right to left, the left condyle must be capable of gliding posteriorly. Since the left condyle is fixed anteriorly, it will not permit translation and you will feel the motion restriction on the right.

You can use the "as if rule" and simply turn your client's head in the direction of the motion restriction and apply pressure to that side in both forward and backward bending to very effectively release the gliding fixations of the occipital condyles. Or you can be more specific in your technique now that you know where the gliding fixations are to be found in flexion and extension. The rules are: in forward bending the anteriorly fixed condyle is on the side opposite to the motion restriction and in backward bending the posteriorly fixed condyle is on the same side as the motion restriction.

If you find a motion restriction in backward bending, just apply the technique outlined above. If you find a motion restriction in forward bending you can vary your technique to directly address the posteriorly fixed condyle. Suppose you find a motion restriction in forward bending while translating from left to right but not from right to left. The right condyle is fixed anteriorly and the occiput cannot sidebend to the left. Hold your client's head in forward bending, and sidebend and rotate it to the left with your left hand. Place your right index and/or middle fingers near the right anteriorly fixed condyle and apply pressure in a posterior superior direction as if you were trying to pry the right condyle from its anteriorly fixed position (Figure 6.6, page 70). Or try laying the radial edge of your left index finger along the base of the occiput and place the tip of your right thumb into the area near the right anteriorly fixed condyle. Apply pressure with your thumb in a posterior superior direction as you sidebend and rotate your client's head to the left (Figure 6.7). You are challenging the facet restriction by turning your client's head left and applying pressure with your right fingers or thumb. Turning your client's head left encourages left sidebending and right rotation and hence posterior glide. Meanwhile, the fingers or thumb of your right hand are clearing the restrictions so that posterior glide can actually occur. As always, just wait for the release, or encourage it a little by gently turning and/or jiggling the head more to the left. Don't forget to follow the dance and always check your results by retesting.

In the next chapter we will turn our attention to the other end of the spine and look at the biomechanics of the sacrum and how to release it from its restrictions.

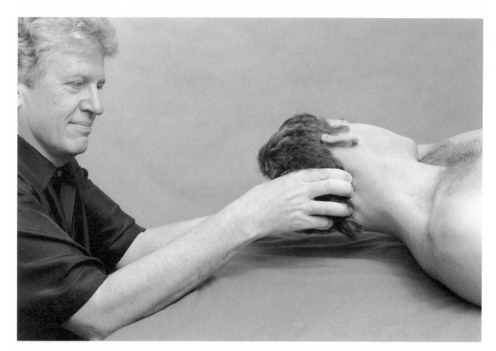

Figure 6.6

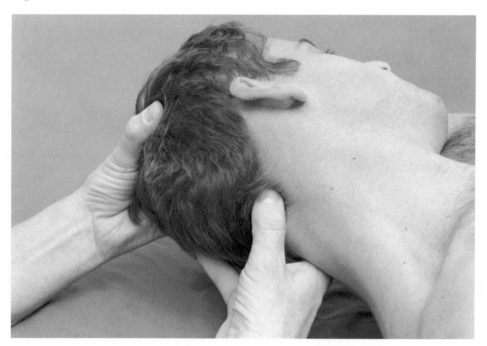

Figure 6.7

7

The Sacrum

THE SACROILIAC JOINT IS INFAMOUS IN ITS REPUTATION FOR CAUSING pain to featherless bipeds. Given the enormous amount of discomfort and pain that is associated with this joint, it is very curious that the word "sacrum" means "the sacred bone."

The sacroiliac (SI) joint is formed by the articulation of the pelvis and the sacrum. Dysfunction of this joint can result from how the pelvis impacts on the sacrum or how the sacrum impacts on the pelvis. If the pelvis is responsible for a fixed SI joint, then it is called a iliosacral dysfunction. If the sacrum is responsible, then it is called a sacroiliac dysfunction. In this chapter you will learn how to recognize and manipulate sacroiliac dysfunctions and in the next you will learn about how to deal with iliosacral dysfunctions.

According to some experts the sacrum is capable of 14 different types of motion. Describing all of these motions can be very interesting, but somewhat tedious unless you just happen to love such activities. My approach in this chapter is to provide a series of quick and easy ways to release the sacrum without first loading you down with complicated biomechanical explanations. We will start our exploration of the sacrum with only the simplest of biomechanical descriptions so that you can begin practicing techniques for releasing the sacrum right away. After your hands are familiar with how the sacrum works, you will learn a more thorough approach to the biomechanics.

Sacral Motion

WHEN YOU FORWARD BEND, YOUR SACRAL BASE MOVES IN A POSTERIOR and slightly superior direction. When you back bend your sacral base moves in the opposite direction, anteriorly and inferiorly. This anterior and posterior movement of the sacrum occurs along a transverse axis that runs through S2. The anterior and posterior movement of the sacral base is called nutation and counternutation, but I will use the simpler designations of anterior nutation and posterior nutation when referring to this motion. The word "nutation" means "nodding."

To find the sacral base on your client, first locate the spinous process of L4. Begin with your client seated in neutral position. With one of your fingers trace an imaginary horizontal line from the crest of the ilium to the spine. The spinous process your finger lands on belongs to L4 (Figure 7.1). Count down to the spinous process of L5 and then one more notch to the sacral base. Or find the sacral base by finding the sacral sulcus (Figure 7.2). The sacral sulcus are vertical grooves that your thumbs will sink into if you roll them just medially off the posterior superior iliac spines (PSIS). Place your right thumb on the right sacral base or sulcus and your left thumb on the left sacral base or sulcus. Ask your client to forward and backward bend while you monitor how the sacral base nutates posteriorly in forward bending and anteriorly in backward bending.

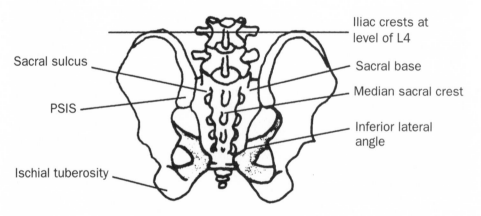

Figure 7.1

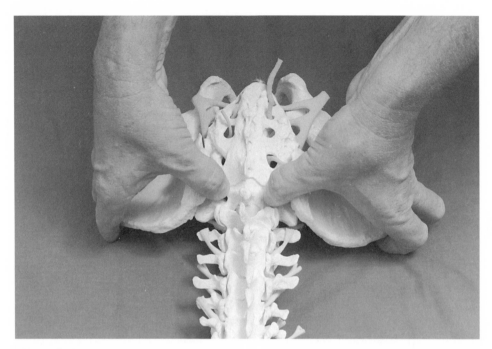

Figure 7.2

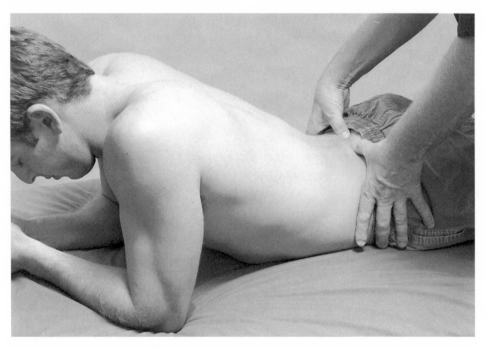

Figure 7.3

It is useful to be able to feel sacral motion in a number of positions so you can double check your results. So ask your client to lay in a prone position on your treatment table. Again place your thumbs on the sacral base. Ask your client to raise himself up and prop himself on his elbows as illustrated in Figure 7.3, page 73, while you feel for whether the sacral base moves anteriorly. Ask your client to lie back down and to then tilt his pelvis posteriorly. This action will accomplish the same results as forward bending. Since most people do not understand what tilting their pelvis posteriorly means, you might suggest that he turn his pelvis under as if to slowly thrust his pubic area forward toward the surface of the table. As he tilts his pelvis posteriorly, feel for whether the sacral base nutates posteriorly. If you do not feel the sacral base nutate either posteriorly or anteriorly, you have discovered a bilateral sacral fixation. Either the sacral base is fixed in bilateral posterior nutation or bilateral anterior nutation.

Sacrums are also capable of sidebending and rotating. If there are no joint fixations, then this is what your sacrum does in walking as you shift your weight from one leg to the other. Most experts agree that the sacrum only exhibits Type I motion and that sidebending and rotation are coupled to opposite sides. Sidebending and rotation of the sacrum are also called torsion. Rotation and torsion of the sacrum are named the same as rotation of the vertebrae. If the right sacral base is posterior, then the sacrum is right rotated or right torsioned (and left sidebent). If the left sacral base is posterior, then the sacrum is left rotated or left torsioned (and right sidebent). It is more accurate but also more complicated to describe rotation and sidebending in terms of torsion but let's leave these complexities for later.

If the sacral base is right rotated in neutral position then it is probably dysfunctional and hence the joint is fixed in some way. Either the right sacral base is fixed in posterior nutation or the left sacral base in fixed in anterior nutation, but how do you determine which side is the fixed side? Forward and backward bend your client and watch how each side behaves.

When your client forward and backward bends, if the rotation of his sacrum appears to go away in forward bending and gets worse in backward bending, then you know that the right side of his sacrum is fixed posteriorly. The right side of the sacrum becomes a fixed point around which the sacrum is forced to turn in forward and backward bending. Since his sacral base is fixed posteriorly, it cannot move anteriorly in backward bending.

So in backward bending his right sacral base stays where it is, posteriorly fixed, while his left sacral base moves further in an anterior direction thereby making it appear that the sacral rotation has worsened. In forward bending his right sacral base again stays where it is, while his left sacral base moves posteriorly, making it appear that the rotation has disappeared.

What happens if your client's sacrum is right rotated, left sidebent, and the left sacral base is fixed anteriorly? His left sacral base in this case will be the fixed pivot point around which his sacrum turns in forward and backward bending. When your client forward bends, his left sacral base stays fixed anteriorly and his right sacral base moves further in a posterior direction and as a result the rotation seems to worsen. When you back bend your client, again his left sacral base remains fixed in its anterior position, but this time his right sacral base moves in an anterior direction, making it seem like the rotation disappears.

Thus, when you find a rotated sacrum, you can create a simple rule for determining which side is fixed. If sacral rotation becomes more extreme in back bending, then the side to which the sacrum is rotated is fixed posteriorly. If sacral rotation seems to disappear in back bending, then the side opposite to the rotation is fixed anteriorly. You can state the rule differently if you wish. I choose to state the rule solely in terms of back bending because so often my evaluation of sacral dysfunction takes place with my client in a prone position on my treatment table. Rather than asking the client to get off the table and sit on the examination stool, it is usually much more convenient and easier to read sacral rotation with him in the prone position. For the sake of practice, however, you should learn to test the sacrum in both the prone and seated positions.

In any case, there are always a number of ways to state these rules. Here is another possibility you might prefer: if the rotation disappears in back bending, then the sacrum is fixed anteriorly on the side opposite its rotation, and if the rotation disappears in forward bending, then the sacrum is fixed posteriorly on the side to which it is rotated.

Techniques

IF PALPATION REVEALS THAT THE SACRUM IS ROTATED, YOU CAN USE A simple indirect technique to derotate it. Recall the first indirect technique that you learned in Chapter One to derotate vertebrae: it can be applied in the same way to the sacrum. With your client in either a seated or prone position, place your thumbs on each side of the sacral base. If his sacrum is left rotated, the left sacral base will be posterior and the right sacral base will be anterior. Push the sacrum further into rotation by increasing the pressure of your right thumb, wait, follow the dance, and let the sacrum derotate itself.

As you already know, this sort of indirect technique does not challenge the facet restriction. As a result, it tends to be a less effective way to release fixations. Before you can challenge a joint fixation, you must know the location of the fixation and whether it is fixed anteriorly or posteriorly. Do this by using the forward and backward bending test in order to determine whether one side is fixed anteriorly or posteriorly.

If the sacrum is right rotated and fixed posteriorly on the right, back bend your client to encourage the right side of his sacrum to move anteriorly and apply several pounds of pressure to his right sacral base in an anterior and slightly inferior direction. Wait for the dance of the tissues and for the release. You can apply this technique with your client in a seated position (Figure 7.3), or with your client prone propped up, and resting on his elbows as a way to back bend and challenge the posteriorly fixed side (Figure 7.4).

If his sacrum is right rotated and fixed anteriorly on the left, forward bend your client to encourage the left side of the sacrum to move posteriorly. Apply several pounds of pressure to his left base in an inferior direction with your thumb. With your other thumb, push the right base, or push further down on the right side, in an anterior direction, as if you were trying to lever the left side free by pushing on the right. Wait for the dance and the release. You can use this technique with your client in a seated position (Figure 7.5, page 78) or prone. In the prone position place a doubled-up pillow under your client's abdomen to forward bend and challenge the anteriorly fixed side and then apply your pressure (Figure 7.6).

If your evaluation of the sacrum reveals that it is bilaterally fixed in posterior nutation, then back bend your client to challenge the bilateral fixation and equally apply several pounds of pressure with your thumbs to each side of his sacral base (Figure 7.7). Apply your pressure in an anterior and slightly inferior direction and wait for the dance and the release.

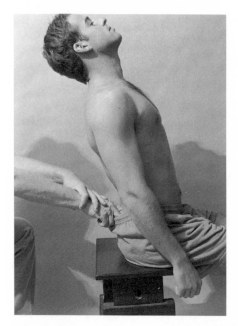

Figure 7.3

You can of course use this technique with your client in either a seated or prone position.

If the sacrum is bilaterally fixed in anterior nutation, forward bend your client to challenge the bilateral fixation and equally apply several pounds of pressure to both sides of his sacral base in an inferior direction (Figure 7.8, page 79). Wait for the dance and for the release. Again you can apply this technique in either the seated or prone position. If you elect to release a sacrum fixed in bilateral anterior nutation, use a doubled-up pillow under your client's abdomen to encourage posterior nutation.

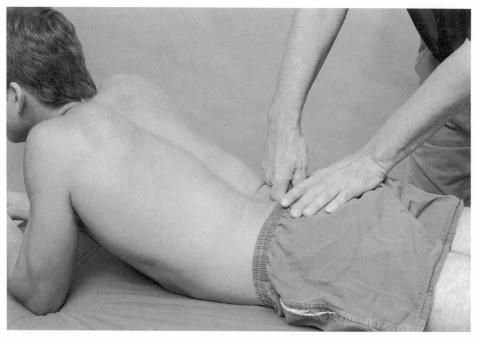

Figure 7.4

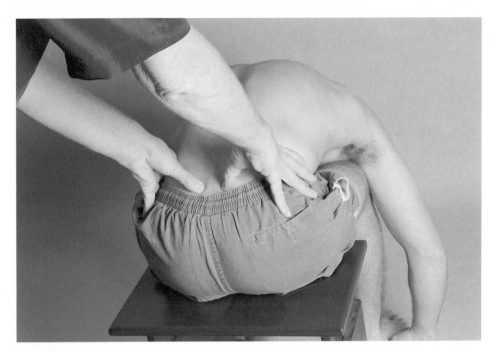

Figures 7.5

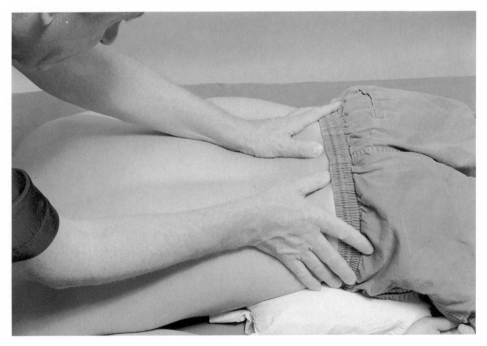

Figure 7.6

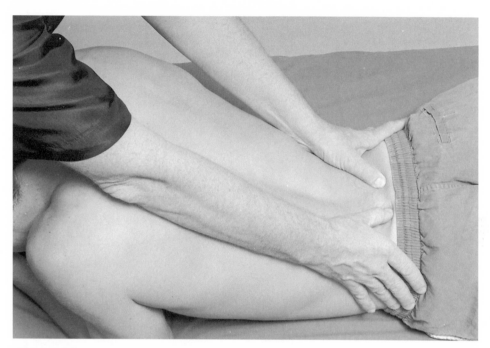

Figures 7.7

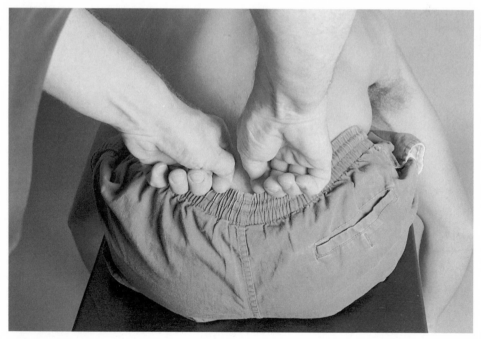

Figure 7.8

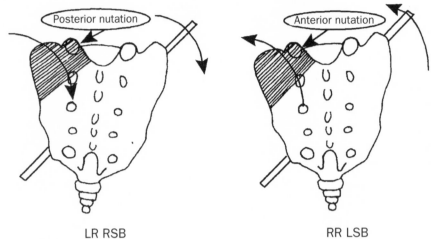

LR RSB
Left torsion (or rotation) on Right axis

RR LSB
Right torsion (or rotation) on Right axis

Figure 7.9

Figure 7.10

Sacral Torsion

Y OU NOW HAVE ENOUGH INFORMATION AND TECHNIQUES TO RELEASE
most sacral dysfunctions. There is another kind of sacral dysfunction
that involves a sacral shear, but before we explore this, let's expand our
understanding of sacral torsion. To some degree you already know what
sacral torsion is, because I introduced it as rotation and sidebending. Introducing torsion as another way to talk about sacral rotation and sidebending will not require learning any new techniques. The techniques remain
the same—only the language changes. You might be tempted to skip this
discussion, but I recommend that you persist because it will help you to
become a more effective therapist.

Sidebending and rotation of the sacrum are called "torsion" which
occurs around either right or left oblique axis. The convention states that
the left oblique axis runs from the superior aspect of the left articulation
of the sacrum on the ilium to the right inferior aspect of the sacrum where
it articulates with the right ilium and the right oblique axis runs from the
superior aspect of the right articulation of the sacrum on the ilium to the
left inferior aspect of the sacrum where it articulates with the left ilium.

The right and left oblique axes and varieties of torsion are shown in
Figures 7.9, 7.10, 7.11, and 7.12. Notice that each of the four kinds of tor-

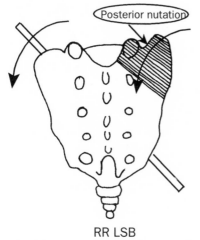

RR LSB
Right torsion (or rotation) on Left axis

Figure 7.11

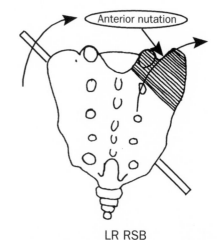

LR RSB
Left torsion (or rotation) on Left axis

Figure 7.12

sion shown is described in terms of the oblique axis on which it is torsioned and as well as in terms of rotation and sidebending. So, for example, Figure 7.12 shows a sacrum in left torsion on the left oblique axis which is also designated as LR and RSB (left rotated and right sidebent). You can correctly say that the sacrum is left rotated on the left oblique axis or left torsioned on the left axis.

Proper body movement while walking is influenced by ability of the sacrum to torsion left on the left axis and right on the right axis. Since most walking is accomplished with your spine relatively upright and vertical, for the purposes of illustration we will assume that your spine and sacrum are in neutral while you walk. You might want to stand and slowly do what is about to be described here so you can get a sense of what happens with your body in normal walking.

As your right leg moves from heel strike to toe off, your body weight begins to move over your right leg, causing your pelvis to shift laterally to the right. As the movement continues toward toe off, your right pelvic innominate bone begins to rotate anteriorly while your left innominate begins to rotate posteriorly. As your right innominate rotates anteriorly, your sacrum moves into right torsion on the right oblique axis (i.e., right rotates and left sidebends because the left sacral base moves in anterior

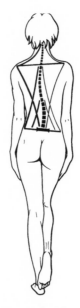

Figure 7.13

nutation). Your lumbar spine sidebends right and rotates left, your thoracic spine sidebends left and rotates right, and your cervical spine sidebends right and rotates right. As the left leg moves from weight bearing to toe off, the left innominate, the sacrum, lumbars, and thoracics torsion, rotate, and sidebend in an opposite manner. Notice in Figure 7.13 how this same complex pattern of pelvic shift, sacral torsion, spinal sidebending, and rotation is introduced as the weight of the body shifts to rest on the left leg. Walking and standing with your weight over one leg introduces and requires this kind of curvature for normal movement.

The way our axial complex alternately undulates in sidebending and rotation as we walk is very interesting and very important to our well-being. Its movement is reminiscent of the vermicular undulation of a snake as it slithers through the grass. The big difference, of course, is that our snake-like spine has been up-ended and given two legs on which to walk. Can you imagine how a snake would be forced to move through its world if we were to snap a number of very tight rubber bands around its body? The resulting dis-ease would spread through its entire but limited experience and body. In an analogous, but more complicated way, joint fixations anywhere along our spine act like the rubber bands around the snake's body. So if at the level of the sacroiliac joint we experience any fixation, whether it is due to pelvis on sacrum or sacrum on pelvis dysfunctions, it can eventually cause trouble throughout our bodies.

So far I have only described neutral sacral torsions—R on R or L on L torsions. When you forward bend and sidebend you introduce non-neutral mechanics into your sacroiliac joint and you create what are called backward or posterior torsions. Take a look at the diagrams (Figures 7.9–7.12) and you will see that in backward or posterior sacral torsions the sacrum either torsions (or rotates) right on the left axis or torsions (or rotates) left on the right axis. Notice that when the sacrum torsions R on L the right sacral base moves posteriorly and when the sacrum torsions L on R the left sacral base moves posteriorly.

Now just as the sacrum can torsion normally in these four ways, it can also get stuck in any one of these ways. So if you find a rotated sacrum when your client is in neutral position, either seated or prone, you can be pretty sure you are looking at a dysfunctional sacrum. In the next chapter on the pelvis you will learn another test to determine sacral dysfunction. It is called the sitting flexion test. But for the time being use rotation as your guide. Then use the forward and back bending tests to determine whether one side is fixed anteriorly or posteriorly. If you discover that the sacral base is fixed anteriorly, it is dysfunctional and you have discovered what is called an anterior sacral torsion. If the sacral base is fixed posteriorly, it is called a posterior sacral torsion. Look once again at the drawings of sacral torsion and notice that there are four ways the sacrum can become dysfunctional in torsion: 1) if the sacrum is torsioned left on the left oblique axis (L on L) and the right sacral base is fixed anteriorly, 2) if the sacrum is torsioned right on the right oblique axis (R on R) and the left base is fixed anteriorly, 3) if the sacral base is torsioned right on the left oblique axis (R on L) and the right sacral base is fixed posteriorly, and 4) if the sacral base is torsioned left on the right oblique axis (L on R) and the left sacral base is posteriorly fixed.

Sacral Shear

THERE IS ONE LAST TYPE OF SACRAL DYSFUNCTION THAT YOU SHOULD know about, called sacral shear. Shear occurs when two surfaces in contact with each other slide on each other in a direction parallel to their plane of contact. Imagine putting two pieces of glass together whose surfaces are wet and pushing them so that they slide on each other. You have just created a shear. Sacral shear is much less common than torsion and its origin, as you probably guessed, is usually traumatic. Sometimes a sacral shear can result from a long-standing lumbar lordosis or a rotoscoliosis in which the lumbar spine curves in odd and unexpected ways.

If you palpate only the sacral base, you cannot distinguish shear from torsion. You might be surprised to know, however, that the techniques you just learned for releasing dysfunctional sacral torsions will also, by and large, release sacral shears, whether you correctly distinguish them from torsions or not. So even if you do not know the difference between shear and torsion, you could unknowingly release a sacral shear, thinking you

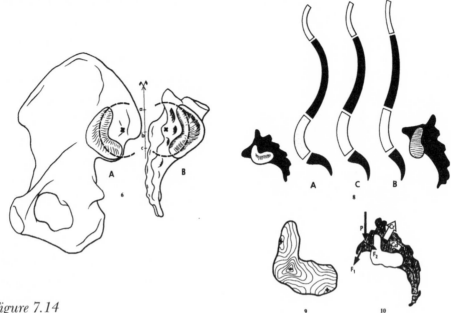

Figure 7.14

are releasing torsion. For the most part, the very same techniques you learned to release torsion will also release shear. Since these techniques do double duty for torsion and shear, you could skip this discussion of sacral shear and still do a lot of good for your clients. But there are some important subtleties that can sometimes make a stunning difference in your effectiveness in dealing with sacral dysfunctions. I will discuss one of these subtleties a little later, because it reveals why the mere mechanical application of technique is not as effective as informed touch.

Figure 7.14 shows quite clearly how the facet of the sacrum fits into a facet on the innominate. The facets are shaped like a fat "L" or "C." Notice how the wide variations in the shape and contour of these facets are correlated to types of spinal curvature. These drawings dramatically demonstrate that any attempt to reposition the sacrum is limited by these inherent shapes and underscores once again the clinical priority of releasing joint restrictions over attempting to reposition bony segments according to some external ideal.

When the sacrum is fixed in a shear the sacral base slips anteriorly or posteriorly around a transverse axis on the facet of the innominate. When

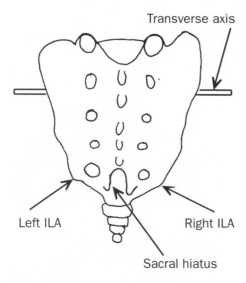

Transverse axis

Left ILA

Right ILA

Sacral hiatus

Figure 7.15

you first palpate the sacral base in a sacrum that has gotten stuck in shear, you will think you are feeling rotation, because one side of the sacral base will be posterior and the other anterior. So you need another reference point on the sacrum to differentiate shear from torsion.

In order to distinguish the two, you palpate the right and left sides of the inferior lateral angle (ILA) of the sacrum. You can find the posterior aspect of the ILA by locating the sacral hiatus. Find the sacral hiatus by running one of your fingers down the center of the sacrum along the spinous processes until your finger lands in the indentation of the sacral hiatus. From the sacral hiatus move your thumbs laterally about one half to three quarters of an inch and you will land on the posterior ILA. The posterior ILA is the transverse process of S5 (Figure 7.15). Let your thumbs slip inferiorly just ever so slightly so that they are resting on the inferior aspect of the ILA and use this aspect of the ILA as your reference point.

Let's imagine that you find a sacrum in which the right base is posterior and the left is anterior. If the sacrum is torsioned, the ILA's will follow the pattern of the torsion and also be posterior on the right and anterior on the left. But if the sacrum is fixed in anterior shear, then the left sacral base will be anterior and the left ILA will be more inferior and posterior than the right ILA. The left ILA also will be more inferior than it is posterior. So in order to distinguish between shear and torsion, you should always palpate not just the sacral base, but also the ILA's. If the left sacral base is anterior and the left ILA is anterior and the right ILA is posterior, then you are looking at a torsion. If the left sacral base is anterior and the left ILA is more inferior and posterior than the right ILA (and more inferior than posterior), then you are looking at a sacral shear.

Anterior sacral shear is much more common than posterior sacral shear. Some think that posterior sacral shear may be no more than just a theoretical possibility, but I have found them and know they exist. So for example, in a right posterior shear of the sacral base, the right sacral base is posterior and the left sacral base is anterior. The right ILA is more superior and anterior than the left ILA and the right ILA will be more superior than it is anterior.

A sacrum fixed in anterior shear is called a unilateral sacral flexion or a unilateral anteriorly nutated sacrum, and a sacrum fixed in posterior shear is called a unilateral sacral extension or a unilateral posteriorly nutated sacrum. But I prefer to call these two fixations anterior and posterior shear of the sacral base. This way of naming shear is a bit clearer, I believe, in that it designates the fixation in the description and therefore immediately tells you where you need to work to facilitate a release. You can call it what you will, of course, but the critical question for you as the therapist is to determine whether the sacral base is fixed in anterior or posterior shear.

First you palpate the sacral base. If you find that one side is posterior and the other is anterior, in order to differentiate shear and torsion you then palpate the ILA's. If palpation of the ILA's reveals shear, your next step is to determine whether the anterior base or the posterior base is the fixed side. Testing for whether the sacral base is fixed in anterior or posterior shear is the same as testing for whether the sacral base is fixed in anterior or posterior sacral torsion. You forward and back bend your client and watch how the sacral base behaves.

Let's look at anterior sacral shear first (Figure 7.16). If the left sacral base is fixed in anterior sacral shear, the left sacral base will be anterior and the right sacral base will be posterior. The left ILA will be more inferior and posterior than the right ILA, and the left ILA will be more inferior than it is posterior. Put your thumbs on each side of the sacral

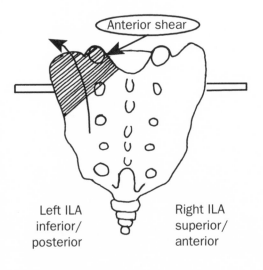

Left ILA
inferior/
posterior

Right ILA
superior/
anterior

Figure 7.16

base and watch what happens in forward and backward bending. Since the left side is fixed in anterior shear, it will become a fixed pivot point around which the right sacral base will be forced to move in forward and backward bending. When you forward bend your client her left sacral base will stay fixed anteriorly and the right sacral base will move in a more posterior direction making the difference between the two sides more extreme. When you backward bend your client her left anterior base remains fixed anteriorly and her right sacral base moves in a more anterior direction, making the difference between the two sides disappear.

Let's look at what happens if your client's right sacral base is fixed in posterior shear (Figure 7.17). Palpation will reveal that her left sacral base is anterior and her right sacral base is posterior. It will also show that the right ILA is more superior and anterior than the left ILA, and the right ILA is more superior than it is anterior. In forward and backward bending her right sacral base becomes the fixed pivot point around which her left sacral base is forced to move. When you backward bend your client, her right sacral base will stay in its posteriorly fixed position and her left sacral base will move more in an anterior direction. As a result, the difference between her two sides will become more extreme. When you forward bend your client her right sacral base maintains its posteriorly fixed position and her left sacral base moves in a more posterior position, making the difference between the two sides disappear.

The forward and back bending test reveals whether the sacral base is fixed anteriorly or posteriorly in exactly the same way for both torsion and shear. Therefore, you can use the same rules we formulated for torsion to help you figure out whether the sacral base is fixed anteriorly or posteriorly in sacral shear. Thus, for example, if the posterior sacral base remains posterior while the anterior side moves anteriorly

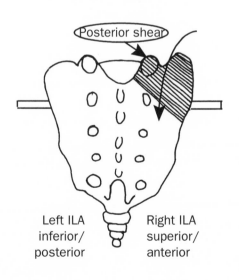

Posterior shear

Left ILA
inferior/
posterior

Right ILA
superior/
anterior

Figure 7.17

during back bending, then the posterior side is fixed in posterior shear. If the anterior sacral base remains anterior while the posterior side moves anteriorly during back bending, then the anterior side is fixed in anterior shear.

The Rumpelstiltskin Effect

IF YOU DO NOT PALPATE THE ILA'S, YOU HAVE NO WAY TO DISTINGUISH between shear and torsion. The same is true if you only use the forward and backward bending tests. Forward and backward bending can only test for which side is fixed anteriorly or posteriorly—it cannot tell you all by itself whether the anterior or posterior fixation it reveals goes with a torsion or a shear. You must palpate the ILA's to determine the difference. Interestingly enough the very same techniques you learned for releasing an anteriorly or posteriorly fixed sacral base in a torsion will also release an anteriorly or posteriorly fixed sacral base associated with shear. The upshot of this discussion is a bit peculiar. If you only palpate the sacral base and use the forward and backward bending tests without palpating the ILA's, and if you only use the joint challenging techniques you learned for releasing sacral torsions, you will also be able to release sacral shear without being aware that it even exists. In practical terms, since the technique is pretty much the same in both cases, it might seem as though knowing how to differentiate shear from torsion is unnecessary.

So you might be wondering why bother learning how to distinguish between shear and torsion in the first place? One answer is that a therapist should just know these things. Another answer is that once you know what these differences are you can add variations to your techniques that will make them more effective in releasing shear. The last answer is harder to understand, but is probably the most significant. Knowing what you are releasing in a client's body adds to your clarity of purpose and actually makes you a more effective therapist. If you know what it is that needs to change, then the techniques you apply will be more effective than if you don't know precisely what you are releasing. This characteristic of the somatic manual arts reminded my wife of the psychotherapeutic setting where, metaphorically, you must name your demons if you want to get rid of them. She calls this phenomenon, "The Rumpelstiltskin Effect."

As strange as it may sound, I am convinced that your recognition of the fixation is more than just an intellectual accomplishment that happens to accompany your application of a technique—it is actually an important part of the technique itself. Before I knew how to tell the difference between shear and torsion, I had developed the techniques described in this chapter for releasing torsion. During the time I was reading about and trying to understand shear, I was working with a client who had what I believed was a posterior torsion in which the right base was posteriorly fixed. For a number of sessions I had applied my technique for posterior torsion. I was able to give him some relief from his pain, but I couldn't get rid of all of it. My client told me at the beginning and end of every session that even though the other pains around his low back area had gone away, the pain in his butt never went away. The pain he was complaining about was in close proximity to the right ILA. I now realize that it is common for clients with sacral shear problems to complain of pain in the area of one of their ILA's, especially in weight bearing situations. When I finally got clear about how to tell the difference between shear and torsion, I palpated my client's ILA's and discovered that he had a right posterior sacral shear. Adding this recognition—that his sacrum was actually in posterior shear, not posterior torsion—to the very *same* technique I had used when I believed his sacrum was posteriorly torsioned fully released his sacrum for the first time. And for the first time the pain in the right side of his buttocks disappeared.

This example is not an isolated case. My experience and the experience of my friends and colleagues has shown us over and over again that knowing and naming what you are working on is an essential part of effective therapy. I have a lot of ideas about why this is so and could lay out what I think is a rather interesting theory about what is happening. But it would require a rather lengthy philosophical discussion that would take us well beyond the scope of this manual. If your understanding is stimulated by poetry, you might appreciate how a line from the great poet, Stefan George, explains how profoundly our lives can be influenced by not knowing the name of something: "Where the name breaks off, no thing may be."

In any case, my observation is very easy to test and would make for an interesting study in somatic manual therapy. Find 20 experienced therapists and 20 patients with sacral shear. Teach 10 therapists how to recognize and treat for sacral torsion only, teach the other 10 therapists how to treat and recognize the difference between shear and torsion, and make sure both groups of therapists learn the same technique for releasing an anterior and posterior sacral base. Then turn them loose on the patients and see what happens.

The most important conclusion for you as a therapist to draw from this discussion is that the clearer you are about what you are working on the more effective you will become. In terms of the techniques you learn from this book, you will find that the simple indirect and shotgun techniques are less effective for the reasons already given earlier, but also because they don't demand the same level of knowledge as the techniques that are specific to the joint fixation. I introduced these simple techniques first as a pedagogical device. Their simplicity is designed to give you a kind of palpatory understanding that prepares the way and makes it easier understanding the more complicated biomechanical descriptions.

If a therapist is more inclined to use these simple indirect and shotgun techniques, it usually means that he doesn't fully grasp the biomechanical descriptions and how to more precisely locate the joint fixation. The biomechanical descriptions are important to your grasp of your client's problem. If a therapist doesn't have this understanding, he won't fully grasp the problem in his client's body. As a result he won't have the same clarity of purpose as the therapist who is oriented toward the specifics of the joint fixation—and without this clarity of purpose, his application of technique will be less effective. If a therapist knows how to locate the joint fixation, she will choose the technique that specifically addresses the problem, because the other method is inefficient and time consuming. But the experienced therapist also picks the more specific approach because at some level she understands the Rumpelstiltskin effect and how powerful clarity of purpose is for effective therapy. This understanding also constitutes part of what I described in the introduction as the healer's way of being.

Variations on Technique

BEFORE WE CONCLUDE THIS CHAPTER ON THE SACRUM, I WANT TO PRESENT some variations on the techniques that you learned for anterior and posterior torsion that make them more specific to anterior and posterior shear. The idea is to help you become more specific and hence more effective in your approach to anterior and posterior shear. You may want to refer to the drawings of the sacrum in anterior and posterior shear (7.16–7.17) as you read through these variations

Recall the technique for manipulating a torsioned sacrum with an anteriorly fixed sacral base. You forward bend your client, put your thumbs on each side of the sacral base, apply pressure in an inferior direction to the anteriorly fixed base, wait for the dance of the tissues, and then the release. Remember that you can further add to your effectiveness if you also add some pressure in an inferior/anterior direction to the opposite sacral base or in an anterior direction to the opposite ILA as a way to lever the anteriorly fixed base in a posterior direction.

Now for the sake of comparison let's say you find a sacral shear in which the left sacral base is fixed anteriorly. You can use pretty much the same technique: ask your client to forward bend and apply pressure in an inferior direction to the left sacral base (Figure 7.18). You can also apply some

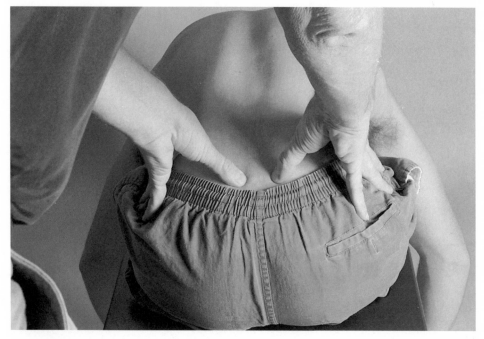

Figure 7.18

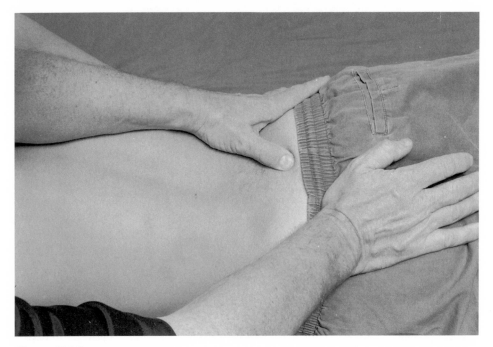

Figure 7.19

anterior pressure to the right sacral base to lever the anterior fixed side in a posterior direction. But make sure you don't use the other variation for anterior torsion in which you apply anterior pressure to the right ILA. It works for left anterior torsion because the right ILA is positioned *posteriorly*. But it won't work for left anterior shear, because the right ILA is positioned superiorly and *anteriorly*. Instead, you could add to your effectiveness by applying pressure to the *right* ILA in an *inferior* direction, as in Figure 7.19, where the client is lying on a doubled-up pillow. Or you could add to your effectiveness by working with the *left* ILA. Since the left ILA is positioned inferiorly and posteriorly, you can facilitate the release of the left sacral base by applying pressure to the left ILA in a superior and anterior direction. So, for example, with your client in a forward bent position (in Figure 7.20 the client is again lying on a doubled-up pillow), you can put one thumb on the left sacral base and the other on the left ILA. With your thumbs positioned in this way you can rock the left side of the sacrum out of its anterior fixation. Alternately push inferiorly on the left sacral base, and superiorly and anteriorly on the left ILA. Rock

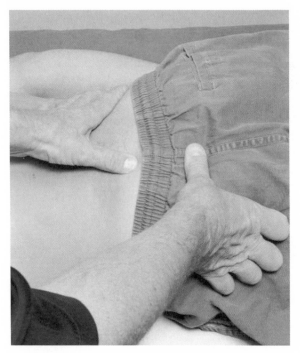

Figure 7.20

the left side of the sacrum in this way in a continuous easy motion, stop, and then apply appropriate pressure to either the left base or the left ILA and wait for the dance and release.

Recall how you manipulate a torsioned sacrum with a posteriorly fixed sacral base. You back bend your client, apply pressure in an anterior direction to the posteriorly fixed base, wait for the dance, and then the release. For comparison, let's suppose you find a sacrum fixed in right posterior shear. You can of course use the same technique for posterior shear that you used for posterior torsion. Or you can further your effectiveness by adding some pressure to the right ILA. Since the right ILA is positioned superiorly and anteriorly, you could push superiorly on the right ILA while you could push anteriorly on the right posteriorly fixed sacral base (Figure 7.21, page 94). Or you can put one thumb on the right posteriorly fixed sacral base and the heel of your other hand on the *left* ILA. Since the left ILA is positioned superiorly and posteriorly, you could push anteriorly and inferiorly on the left ILA while you push anteriorly on the right sacral base (Figure 7.22).

Once you have a clear understanding of the type of fixation you are dealing with and the ways the sacrum can be positioned, then you can make up your own techniques and variations.

In this chapter you learned how to recognize and manipulate sacroiliac dysfunctions that were caused by eight different sacral fixations. In the next you will learn how to recognize and release fixations that are created by the pelvis.

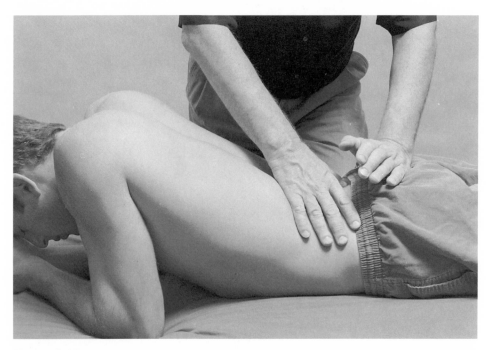

Figure 7.21

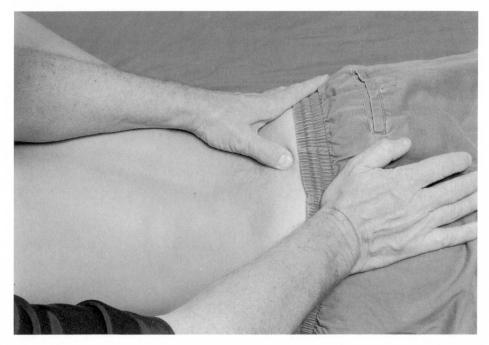

Figure 7.22

8

The Pelvis

THE SACRUM AND THE PELVIS ARE SO CLOSELY TIED TOGETHER THAT when they exist freely in their natural state of cooperative independence life can be grand. But when one or the other interferes with normal motion, pain and misery can descend quickly, like a black cloud capable of obscuring even the best of our shining moments. You already know the ways the sacrum can create painful problems in this area. The influence of the pelvis on the sacroiliac (SI) joint can be just as problematic. Knowing how to recognize and treat the many dysfunctions caused by the pelvis is extremely important if you want to be able to resolve your client's low back pain. If you do a great job of releasing your client's sacrum, but do not take care of its interaction with the pelvis, much of your work will be in vain. If you do not release iliosacral (pelvis on sacrum) fixations, it will not be long before most, if not all, of your client's pain returns.

Like every area of the body you decide to study, the pelvic area is very complicated and interconnected to the rest of the body. In this chapter you will be learning primarily about joint dysfunction, but you also want to appreciate the intimate connections that exist between the pelvis, sacrum, spine, and the rest of the body. When you study Figure 8.1, page 96, showing the iliosacral and sacroiliac ligaments, you can clearly see how tightly connected the pelvis, sacrum, L4, and L5 are. Whenever you work on any of these structures, remember how they are connected and be certain that you have released all the associated restrictions. As you are about

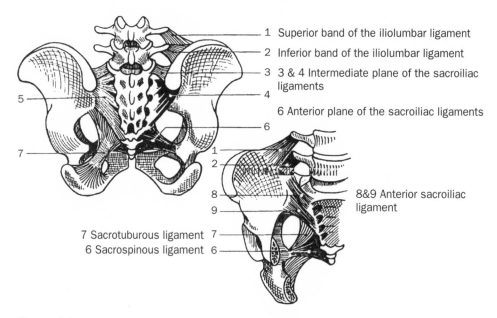

1 Superior band of the iliolumbar ligament

2 Inferior band of the iliolumbar ligament

3 3 & 4 Intermediate plane of the sacroiliac ligaments

6 Anterior plane of the sacroiliac ligaments

8&9 Anterior sacroiliac ligament

7 Sacrotuburous ligament

6 Sacrospinous ligament

Figure 8.1

to learn, the pelvis can cause problems in three ways. Any one or combination of these patterns of pelvic dysfunction will also strain the ligaments and create further dysfunction in the low back and sacrum.

Be aware that the iliolumbar, sacrospinous, and sacrotuberous ligaments are three very important ligaments in this area. Along with the pelvic rotaters (especially the piriformis) and the psoas, they must be capable of adapting to your manipulations in order to create long lasting change for your clients. You probably already have your favorite ways of releasing these muscles and ligaments. Make sure you address them either before or after releasing all sacroiliac or iliosacral fixations.

Ligamentous structures are clearly important for proper joint function, but so is overall body structure and posture. The alignment of your body in gravity can profoundly affect how your pelvis is positioned and this in turn can determine how well your joints function. The drawings in Figure 8.2 represent four ways the pelvis can be positioned with respect to the entire body. " Tilt" refers to the anterior or posterior torsioning of the entire pelvis around a transverse axis that runs through the inferior aspect of the sacroiliac joint. "Shift" refers to the anterior or posterior

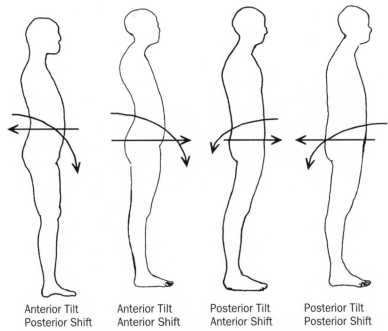

Anterior Tilt	Anterior Tilt	Posterior Tilt	Posterior Tilt
Posterior Shift	Anterior Shift	Anterior Shift	Posterior Shift

Figure 8.2   TILT occurs as an anterior or posterior torsioning of the entire pelvis around a transverse axis that runs through the inferior aspect of the sacroiliac joint.
SHIFT occurs as an anterior or posterior translation of the entire pelvis along the transverse plane.

translation of the entire pelvis along the transverse plane. The curved arrows represent tilt and the straight arrows indicate shift. The difference between tilt and shift was first recognized by Jan Sultan and is part of a brilliant typology he developed for identifying common structural types and their associated myofascial strain and gait patterns. His understanding of tilt/shift was further refined by Swiss Rolfer, Dr. Hans Flury.

Many myofascial structures contribute to these overall patterns. For example, a posteriorly tilted pelvis is often tied to tight, short hamstrings while an anteriorly tilted pelvis is often tied to tight, short quadriceps. These postural issues are also often associated with typical sacral dysfunctions. When the sacrum gets stuck bilaterally in posterior nutation it often drags the lumbars with it, especially L4 and L5. As it turns out, a person whose pelvis inclines toward posterior tilt will more likely show bilateral posterior nutation fixations of the sacrum than a person with an anterior pelvis.

Not recognizing the difference between tilt and shift has mislead many

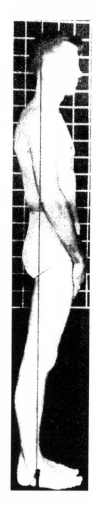

Figure 8.3

therapists in their evaluations of clients' overall alignment. When a client's pelvis is posteriorly tilted, but shows an anterior shift well beyond the mid-sagittal axis, it is common to misread this pattern as a lordosis or a swayback. As the pelvis shifts anteriorly, the thorax shifts posteriorly giving the person the appearance of falling backward. But if you look carefully, you will often see a lumbar spine that is actually lacking an appropriate lordosis. The illusion of a swayback is created by an anterior shift of the pelvis. Figure 8.3 is from Kendall and McCreary's *Muscles: Testing and Function*[1] and is a clear case of an anteriorly shifted pelvis with a posterior tilt. Notice that this person's lumbar spine is actually rather flat and displays very little lordotic curve. Although this example is not extreme, clearly Kendall and McCreary are misled by the anterior shift of a posteriorly tilted pelvis and wrongly describe this person as having a swayback posture. This pattern of the anterior shift of a posteriorly tilted pelvis can be slight for one person and very extreme in another, but in most cases you will see that the lordotic curve is lacking to some degree.

Although dealing with these many and varied postural issues is well beyond the scope of this manual, some discussion is helpful. It serves to remind you of the of importance of always trying to understand how local fixations are intimately related to whole body structure and gravity. In a very real sense, you can never work on any local area of the body without being in contact with the whole body and its complicated network of compensations. If a local change is introduced into a body without taking account of its network of compensations and postural habits, then typically the body will not be able to sustain the change. If it cannot adapt above or support the change below, then either the body will return to its original dysfunction or develop strain and dysfunction elsewhere—or both.

Testing and Palpating for Iliosacral Dysfunction

Let's leave these larger issues and turn our attention to the specifics of how the pelvis creates joint fixations. The three ways the pelvis can create dysfunction are torsion, flare, and shear. First you will learn what these patterns are and then you will learn how to test and release them. You have already encountered pelvic torsion in the last chapter where I described the vermicular undulation of the spine during walking. You may recall how normal walking requires that each innominate rotate (or torsion) anteriorly and posteriorly in response to how each leg moves from heel strike to toe off. Torsion of the innominates occurs around a transverse axis that runs through the inferior aspect of the sacroiliac joint. Just as it is possible for the innominates to torsion normally, it is also possible for one of them to get stuck in either anterior or posterior torsion.

Flare of the innominate can occur as either out-flare or in-flare. When out-flared, the ilium rotates laterally, or away from the mid-sagittal axis as the ischial tuberosity rotates medially, or toward the mid-sagittal axis. In-flare behaves in the opposite fashion: the ilium rotates medially toward the mid-sagittal axis and the tuberosity rotates away from the mid-sagittal axis.

Shear is a just a bit more complicated, because it can occur in two distinct ways, either as anterior/posterior shear or superior/inferior shear. In superior/inferior shear, also known as up-slip and down-slip, one of the innominates either slips upward on the sacrum in relation to the other innominate or it slips downward. In anterior/posterior (A/P) shear, one of the innominates either slips anteriorly in relation to the other innominates or it slips posteriorly. You could reasonably call A/P shear anterior and posterior slip.

You are probably wondering how you determine whether a client is manifesting one of these iliosacral fixations and, if she is, how you tell whether the innominate is fixed anteriorly or posteriorly or inferiorly or superiorly. As you might have guessed, the osteopaths have created some rather simple tests to help you answer these questions.

The first test for determining iliosacral dysfunction is the standing flexion test. To perform it you need to place your thumbs on the inferior

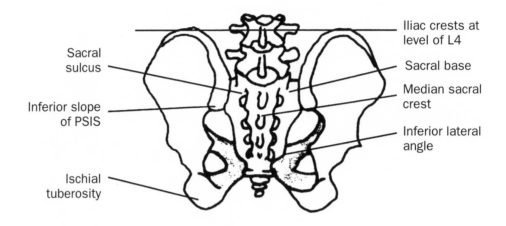

Sacral sulcus

Inferior slope of PSIS

Ischial tuberosity

Iliac crests at level of L4

Sacral base

Median sacral crest

Inferior lateral angle

Figure 8.4

slopes of the posterior superior iliac spines (PSIS), illustrated in Figure 8.4. You can find the PSIS by looking for the dimples most people have in this area, located about two inches lateral to the lumbosacral junction. By placing the pads of your thumbs over them you will find the most posterior aspect of the PSIS. Drag your thumbs in an inferior direction until you find the inferior slopes of the PSIS. You will know you are there when you feel your thumbs just begin to slide off the inferior aspect of the PSIS.

With your client standing, place the pads of your thumbs on the inferior slope of the PSIS and ask him to bend forward as far as he comfortably can. Watch what happens to your thumbs. If there is an iliosacral fixation, one of your thumbs will ride up in a superior direction and the other one will stay where it is. The side on which the thumb rides up is the fixed side. Figure 8.5 shows the restriction on the right side. This test works quite well, unless the hamstrings or the quadratus lumborum are asymmetrically tight. If the hamstrings are tight on the side opposite to where your thumb rides up, or if the quadratus lumborum is tight on the same side as where your thumb rides up, the superior movement of your thumb will not be a true indicator.

The standing flexion test will not tell you whether one innominate is

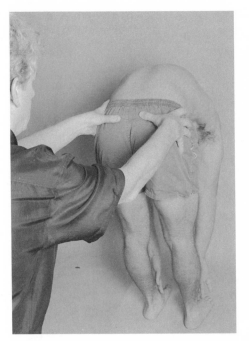

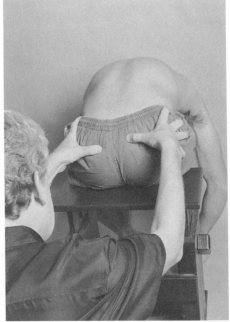

Figure 8.5   *Figure 8.6*

in-flared or out-flared, whether one innominate is up-slipped or down-slipped, whether one is anteriorly slipped or posteriorly slipped, or whether one is posteriorly torsioned or anteriorly torsioned. The tests will only tell you the side on which the innominate is fixed on the sacrum. In order to tell what kind of iliosacral fixation you are looking at you must palpate a number of other areas on the pelvis, a technique that will be described shortly. For now, just practice the standing flexion test and notice what happens to your thumbs.

Now that you have learned how to use this test to determine iliosacral dysfunction, you can use the sitting version of it to help you determine unilateral sacroiliac fixations. Ask your client to assume a seated position, once again place the pads of your thumbs on the inferior slope of the PSIS, and ask him to forward bend as far as he comfortably can. If one of your thumbs rides superiorly, as it does in Figure 8.6, you have discovered a sacroiliac fixation. Like the standing flexion test, the sitting flexion test only tells you on which the side the sacral fixation exists, it doesn't tell whether it is fixed in anterior/posterior torsion or anterior/posterior shear.

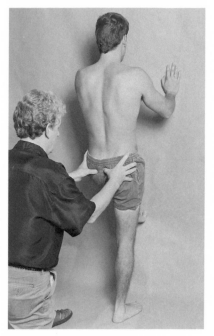

Figure 8.7

The sitting flexion test effectively removes the influence of your client's legs and pelvis on the sacrum and therefore allows you to determine whether sacroiliac fixations are present. In contrast, the standing flexion test adds the influence of the pelvis and legs, and lets you determine whether iliosacral fixations are present. If your thumb rides up in both the sitting and standing flexion tests, then you have discovered a sacroiliac and iliosacral dysfunction. Knowing how to use these tests is helpful to sorting out what kind of fixations are present.

Often you may be working with clients whose low back problems create too much pain when they try to forward bend from a standing position. In these cases, and as a way to double check your results, the so-called stork test is also very useful. Ask your client to stand facing a wall so he can stabilize himself while performing the test. Put the pad of your right thumb on the posterior aspect of his right PSIS and your left thumb at the same level on the median sacral crest, which is basically the mid-line of the sacrum. Ask your client to raise his knee to at least 90 degrees and watch what your right thumb does (Figure 8.7). If there is no iliosacral fixation, your right thumb will ride inferiorly as he raises his leg and your left thumb will remain where it is. If there is a fixation, then your right thumb will remain where it is and not move inferiorly. Test the other side in the same way. Place your left thumb on the posterior aspect of his left PSIS and your right thumb at the same level on the medial sacral crest, ask him to raise his knee to at least 90 degrees, and watch how your left thumb responds. If it doesn't move inferiorly, you have discovered an iliosacral fixation.

If either the standing flexion or the stork test reveals an iliosacral fixation, the next part of your evaluation requires you to figure out by means of palpation whether you are dealing with flare, shear, torsion, or a combination of some or all of them. Let's take a simplified look at an example. Suppose you find an iliosacral fixation on the right by using the standing flexion test, and you palpate the innominates to discover that the right innominate seems out-flared and the left seems in-flared. If you had palpated the innominates without having performed the standing flexion test, it would be very difficult for you to be able to say whether the right innominate was out-flared or the left innominate was in-flared. But since you performed the standing flexion test and it revealed that the fixation was on the right, you can conclude that the right innominate must be fixed in an out-flared position. So here is how it works: first you determine the side on which the fixation is present; then you palpate to determine whether the iliosacral fixation is an in-flare or out-flare, an anterior or posterior shear, an up-slip or down-slip, an anterior or posterior torsion, or some combination.

Palpating for In-flare/Out-flare

Let's look more carefully at where and how you palpate for each of these conditions. We will begin with palpating for in-flare and out-flare. Find the anterior superior iliac spine (ASIS) (Figure 8.8) with your client in a supine position. The easiest way to do this is to first place your palms over the ASIS to locate it and notice how the shape of this area feels to your touch. Then place the pads of your thumbs on the medial inferior edge of each ASIS. Next draw an imaginary line down the center of your client's body to represent the mid-sagittal axis. On most people the navel is on this center line. Then compare how far each thumb is from this center line. If the thumb on the right ASIS seems closer to the midline than the left, then you are probably looking at an unilateral in-flare or out-flare. If the standing flexion test or the stork

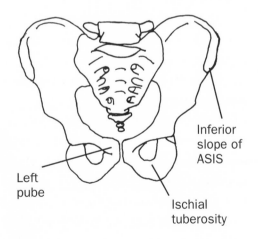

Inferior
slope of
ASIS

Left
pube

Ischial
tuberosity

Figure 8.8

test reveals a fixation on the right, then you have discovered a right in-flare. If the tests show that the fixation is on the left, then you have found a left out-flare.

Palpating for Up-slip/Down-slip (Superior/Inferior Shear)

Shear is most often the result of trauma and although down-slips do occur, they are very rare. When one does occur it is usually corrected by walking. So if your palpation reveals one innominate that seems inferior and one that seems superior, you can pretty much be assured that you are looking at up-slip. Begin your palpation sequence with your client in a prone position. Be sure that your thumbs are always placed on exactly the same level. Place the pads of your thumbs on each of the ischial tuberosities and compare their relative positions to one another. Does one seem superior and the other inferior? If so, and the standing flexion and stork tests show a fixation on the same side as the superior tuberosity, then you have probably discovered an up-slip. The position of the tuberosities is a fairly reliable indicator, but you can be misled under certain circumstances. Sometimes what appears to be an up-slip is the result of curvature in which the lumbar spine sidebends to the same side as the apparent up-slip. A Type I group curvature with a right sidebending, for example, will make the right innominate seem more superior than the left.

Next palpate the PSIS's for their relative superior/inferior positions and then roll your client over and palpate the ASIS's. If the ASIS and PSIS of one of the innominates are both superior, then you are probably looking at an up-slip. Ask your client to return to a prone position and check the sacrotuberous ligaments. To find these ligaments, place your thumbs between the apex of the sacrum and the ischial tuberosities. The sacrotuberous ligament will be lax on the same side as the up-slip and tight on the same side as the down-slip. Ask your client to turn over again and in a supine position palpate the superior edges of the pubes to see if they seem superior and inferior with respect to each other. Lastly check the inguinal ligaments for tenderness. The inguinal ligament will likely be tender on the same side as shear: if it's a right up-slip, it will be tender on the right, and if it's a left down-slip, tender on the left. Be aware that tenderness is a less reliable indicator than position. If the standing flexion and stork tests reveal a fixation on the right and all palpatory indicators show the right side superior in relation to the left, you have discovered a right up-slip.

Palpating for Anterior/Posterior Shear

With your client in a supine position place the pads of your thumbs on the most anterior aspect of each pube and evaluate for whether one seems anterior and the other posterior. If the standing flexion and stork tests reveals a fixation on the right and the right pube is anterior, then the right innominate is fixed in anterior shear. If the tests reveal the fixation on the left, then the left innominate is fixed in posterior shear.

Palpating for Anterior/Posterior Torsion

I left torsion for last because of all the forms of dysfunction we have discussed, it is usually the least likely type of pelvic dysfunction. So, I suggest that in your palpation sequence you also save torsion for last. If you find a shear or flare fixation correct them first before you even palpate for torsion. Almost everybody's innominates torsion in the same way. The normal and expected pattern you will see over and over again is the right innominate torsioned anteriorly and the left posteriorly. If you find the opposite situation you may be looking at trauma, or a soccer player who kicks with his left foot. If the standing flexion test and the stork tests reveal an iliosacral fixation and you palpate torsion first you will predictably find the right innominate torsioned anteriorly and the left posteriorly. More than likely the torsion is normal and the fixation the test revealed is due to shear or flare. So your best bet is to palpate for shear and flare first, correct what you find, and perform the standing flexion and stork tests to check your results. If the fixation is no longer present, there is no need to bother yourself with palpating for torsion. If the fixation persists after correcting shear and flare, then correct for torsion. But if you palpate for torsion before you palpate for flare or shear, you may be mislead into correcting a torsion fixation when none is present.

Palpate for torsion with your client in a supine position. Place your thumbs on the ASIS's and compare their relative positions to one another. Does one innominate seem torsioned anteriorly and the other posteriorly? Let's assume that either you have already released flare or shear dysfunctions or none are present. If the standing flexion and stork tests show a fixation on the right and the right innominate is torsioned anteriorly, then the right innominate is fixed in anterior torsion. If you discover the fixation on the left and the left innominate is torsioned posteriorly, then the left innominate is fixed in posterior torsion.

I have never worked with a client who showed all three iliosacral fixations at once, but I believe it is possible. Often, however, you will find a combination of two of these fixations. Depending on the uniqueness of each client's body, sometimes it is very easy to palpate these patterns and other times it is more difficult. Don't be discouraged if at first you are not quite sure what pattern you looking at. If you are not certain, correct for what you think the problem is and retest. The techniques described in this book for releasing iliosacral fixations are gentle enough that they will not cause harm if you misread the position of the innominate and correct for a problem that is not present. If the standing flexion and stork tests show a fixation and you are unclear from palpation whether you are looking at shear or flare, correct for both on the side on which the fixation shows up. For instance, correct for shear and then retest and, If the test is negative you know the problem was shear. If the test is still positive, correct for flare and retest again. Always palpate before and after manipulation so that you learn to see and feel subtle but important differences. And in time you will learn to see and feel more and more subtle patterns.

Techniques for Pelvis-on-Sacrum Dysfunctions

ALL OF THE TECHNIQUES YOU ARE ABOUT TO LEARN WORK BEST IF YOU free up all the associated soft tissues and ligaments in this area. For example, be sure that the hamstrings, gluteals, rotators, psoas, quadratus lumborum, errectors, and ligaments are balanced and free enough for your client's pelvis to accept pelvic manipulations.

Out-flare

Put your client in a supine position. On the out-flared side bring one of your client's knees up (foot flat on the table). Sit on the same side of the table as the out-flare. Place the fingers of one hand on the medial surface of the ischial tuberosity and the heel of the other hand on the ilium with fingers wrapped around the ASIS (Figures 8.9 and 8.10). Gently but firmly

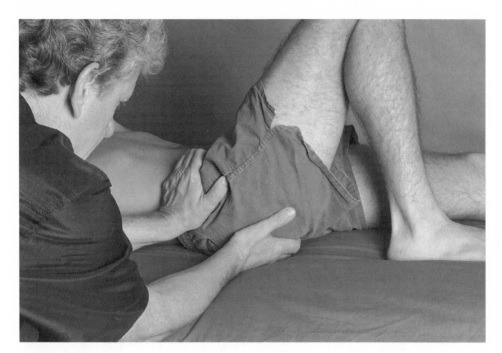

Figure 8.9

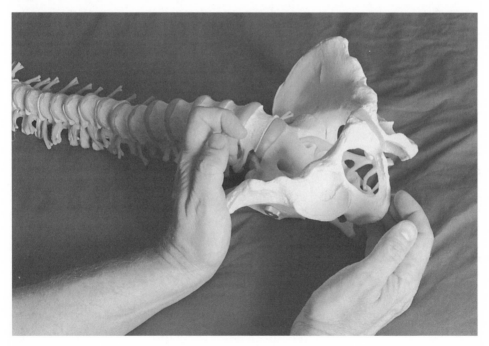

Figure 8.10

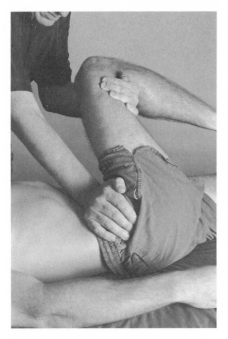

Figure 8.11

traction the tuberosity laterally while pushing the ilium medially and wait. Either the innominate will release its restriction by going through a dance or by moving directly to its normal position. This technique was created by Jan Sultan.

In-flare

Place your client in a supine position and stand on the opposite side of the table from the in-flare. As shown in Figure 8.11, reach across to the knee of the in-flared side. Bend the knee, hook your arm underneath, lift, and bring it across the midline as you pull it in a superior direction. As you hold the knee in this position, pull it toward you ever so slightly to stabilize the tuberosity. Put the heel of your other hand just medial to the ASIS and gently but firmly push the ilium laterally and wait. Either the innominate will go through its dance and release or it will move directly to its normal position.

Up-slip

With your client lying on the side opposite the up-slip, use the leg of the up-slipped side as a handle to guide the innominate. Using the direct technique you gently but firmly pull the leg inferiorly and wait for the innominate to glide into its normal position (Figure 8.12). The indirect technique requires a few more steps. Use the femur to gently but firmly and slowly push the innominate superiorly and hence further into its up-slip. Wait. You will feel the innominate move further into the up-slip. Next you may feel a pulsation and then an impulse in the client's body for the innominate to move inferiorly. When you feel the impulse to move inferiorly, encourage that movement by slowly and gently pulling the leg inferiorly at a speed that matches the speed with which the client's body releases. If

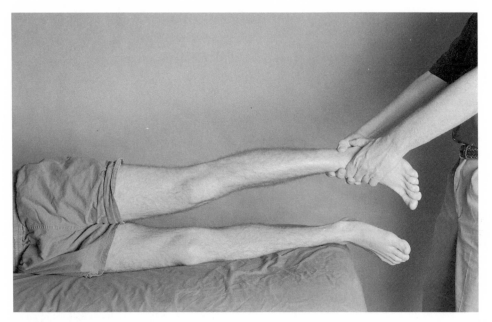

Figure 8.12

at first you are unable to feel the impulse of the body to move inferiorly, don't worry about it. Perform the technique as directed: use the femur to push the innominate further into its up-slip, and simply hold it in that position for about 5 to 10 seconds, and then traction the leg and pelvis inferiorly. These two methods for releasing an up-slip were also created by Jan Sultan.

Down-slip

Simply reverse the direct and indirect up-slip technique. You can use your client's leg to directly push the pelvis superiorly. Or you can pull your client's leg inferiorly to increase the down-slip and wait for the impulse to release superiorly.

Anterior Shear

With your client prone, stand on the same side of the table as the anterior shear. Place the fingers of one hand on the anterior pube and place the forearm of your other arm on the opposite innominate. With your forearm, stabilize the pelvis while you gently but firmly push the anterior

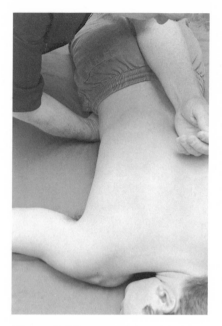

Figure 8.13

pube in a posterior direction (Figure 8.13) and wait. Either the innominate will dance to its release or it will move directly to its normal position.

Posterior Shear

With your client prone, stand on the opposite side of the posterior shear. Use the same hand and forearm placement as described for the anterior shear, but this time use your fingers to stabilize the pube while you use your forearm to gently but firmly push the opposite innominate (with the posterior pube) in an anterior direction. Wait. Either the innominate will release its restriction by dancing this way and that or by moving directly to its normal position.

Anterior Torsion

With your client supine, stand on the same side as the anterior torsion and place the heel of one hand on the ASIS of the anteriorly torsioned innominate (Figure 8.14). Bring the femur perpendicular to the table with the knee bent and lean a little of your body weight on the knee. With your other hand, gently but firmly apply pressure on the ASIS in the direction of posterior torsion as you use your body weight to move the femur to encourage the posterior torsioning of the innominate and wait. Either the innominate will go through its dance or it will move directly to its normal position.

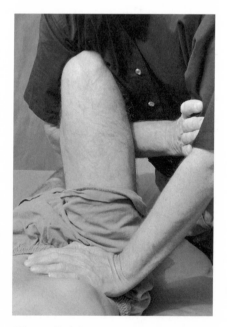

Figure 8.14

110

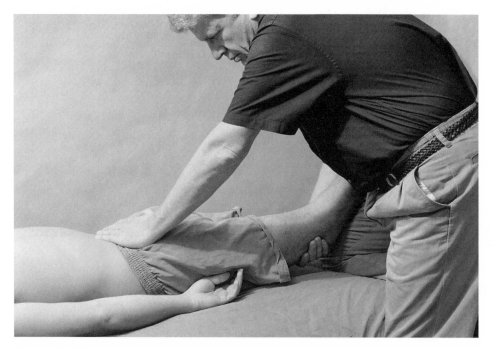

Figure 8.15

Posterior Torsion

With your client prone, stand on the side with the posterior torsion. Place one hand under the femur just above the knee of the posteriorly torsioned innominate and the other hand on the posterior aspect of the innominate itself. Lift the femur slightly off the table and place your knee under it so you don't have to hold the leg up as you perform the technique (Figure 8.15). Gently but firmly apply pressure to the innominate with the other hand in the direction of an anterior torsion and wait. Either the innominate will release its restriction by unwinding or by moving directly to its normal position.

As a general rule, remember that these iliosacral techniques, as well as all the other techniques discussed in this book, work best if you prepare the myofascial and ligamentous tissues associated with the fixations you are attempting to release. Preparing the tissues means that you release the associated strain patterns and bring enough balance to the appropriate areas of your client's body so that he is able to adapt to your manipulations. It also helps if you are able to address the alignment of the whole body along with its many patterns of compensation. As a somatic practitioner you already have your favorite ways of releasing and balancing these tissues, and your techniques are certainly a useful adjunct to the techniques you learn from this book. However, even if you do nothing to prepare the tissues or address patterns of compensation, the techniques taught in this book are still powerful enough to get good results all by themselves.

Note

1. Kendall, Florence Peterson and McCreary, Elizabeth Kendall. *Muscles: Testing and Function.* Third edition, Baltimore: (Williams and Wilkins), 1983.

9

The Ribs

I N THE LAST CHAPTER YOU LEARNED HOW THE PELVIS CONTRIBUTES TO back pain. In this chapter you will learn how the ribs contribute to and help perpetuate back pain. The organization of the thorax, as well as its myofascial, ligamentous, and articular fixations, can profoundly affect the organization, integrity, and functioning of the whole body. If you consider only the joints of the thorax, there are 150 articulations, and most ribs can be involved in 6 articulations alone. Just by freeing a myriad of thoracic restrictions, which might include rib fixations in the ribs, sternum, clavicles, the ligaments and fascia from which the lungs are suspended, and so on, it is sometimes possible to release neck and low back facet restrictions without ever even working on the neck or lower back themselves. In this chapter, however, we will limit our discussion to the ribs only. Once you learn how to recognize and release rib dysfunctions, you will be surprised and pleased at how this knowledge will contribute greatly to your ability to release many facet restrictions in the thoracic and cervical spines.

The Influence of the Ribs

S INCE THE RIBS ARTICULATE WITH THE SPINE IN VERY SPECIFIC WAYS, they play a significant role in spinal dysfunction. Rib 1 articulates with T1 and ribs 11 and 12 articulate with T11 and T12 respectively. Ribs 1, 11, and 12 articulate with the spine by means of unifacets, whereas ribs 2–10 articulate by means of demifacets. All the ribs, with the exception of 11 and 12, articulate in the front of the thorax by means of strong cartilaginous attachments and this cartilage in turn also articulates with the sternum. Look at the front of the thorax and you will see that there are really two attachments, called the costochondral and sternochondral junctions, that are associated with most of these ribs. The costochondral junction acts like a joint and is formed by the insertion of the concave end of the rib into a cone-shaped piece of cartilage. The sternochondral articulation is formed by the costal cartilage inserting into the triangular notches of the sternum, in which are found small synovial joints. Motion occurs at both of these articulations and releasing a rib requires addressing the costochondral junction and sometimes the sternochondral articulations as well.

The complex relation between the ribs and vertebrae illustrated in Figure 9.1 shows why dysfunctional rib torsions usually result from vertebral rotations and Type II dysfunctions in the thoracic spine. The ribs that connect to the spine by means of demifacets articulate with two vertebrae.

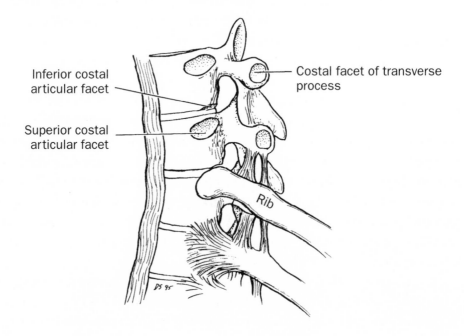

Figure 9.1

Let's look at the fifth rib as an example. Rib 5 attaches to the inferior costal facet of T4, the superior costal facet of T5, and the costal facet of the transverse process of T5. If T4 rotates right on T5, T4 pulls the superior aspect of the rib with it, while the inferior aspect of the rib, which is attached to T5, remains unaffected by the rotation. The right rotation of T4 will thus cause the right fifth rib to torsion externally and the left fifth rib to torsion internally.

Ribs that articulate by means of demifacets have two costovertebral connections and one costotransverse connection. The floating ribs, 11 and 12, which attach by means of a unifacet do not have a costotranverse articulation. Even though they do not attach to the front of the rib cage itself, they do have interesting connections to the muscles of the posterior abdominal wall. These connections are important, because when the articulations of ribs 11 or 12 are fixed, they are accompanied by myofascial strain patterns in the abdominal muscles. As my colleague and friend Jan Sultan discovered, these strain patterns are often in the form of a vortex and they must also be released if you want to successfully release these ribs as well. The ribs even have a tough little ligament that attaches to the annulus of the intervertebral disk. All of these connections mean that a rib in trouble can often cause more pain than a dysfunctional vertebra and learning how to release rib fixations will contribute greatly to your skills.

Due to the intimate relationships between ribs and spine, you can often release rib dysfunctions simply by releasing the vertebral dysfunctions. So the best strategy is to release Type II fixations first. But many times releasing the dysfunctional thoracic vertebra will not be enough to release the rib. So always test and retest both vertebral and rib fixations to make sure your manipulations are successful. Just remember that releasing Type II fixations will sometimes release the rib and sometimes not. Be aware that it also works the other way—Type II fixations will not always remain released until the rib fixations are released.

If you successfully release a dysfunctional thoracic vertebra, your client will probably immediately report feeling better. But if you don't release the associated rib fixation, you can expect to hear how the pain returned within a few hours or days. Sometimes this report means that the unresolved rib fixation was enough to make the facet restriction reassert itself.

And other times it means that your client is still in pain because of the unresolved rib fixations, even though your release of the vertebral dysfunction was completely successful. Ribs are very important in perpetuating back and neck pain. Many cervical fixations are held and maintained by upper rib fixations. I have seen too many clients who received treatments from therapists who knew how to release vertebral dysfunctions, but did not know how to release rib fixations. The result of only releasing the thoracic vertebrae is that often the rib fixations worsen and the client ends up with more pain than before she started treatment. So always check for and release rib fixations. Your clients will love you for it.

Finding the Fixed Ribs

RIBS CAN GET INTO TROUBLE IN A NUMBER OF WAYS. THEY CAN TORSION internally or externally, they can sublux anteriorly or posteriorly, the first rib can slip superiorly, and they can become distorted and dysfunctional through trauma. We will explore how to understand and treat torsion, subluxation, and first rib dysfunction.

The technique for releasing the ribs is very simple and straightforward. All you need to know is how to locate the fixed rib. There are two simple ways to locate a fixed rib that do not require you to know whether the rib is torsioned or subluxed. Once you locate the fixed rib, applying the technique will tell you how the rib is positioned as you follow how it dances toward its release—evaluation and treatment merge together as one and the same process.

Notice that there are two grooves associated with the spine. The spinal groove is between the spinous and transverse processes of the spine. Another groove is formed where the ribs articulate with the spine at the costotransverse junction. Illustrated by the drawing in Figure 9.2, this articulation is roughly at the lateral borders of the errectors. To find this rib groove, place the pad of your thumb on the spinous process, and drag your thumb laterally. Almost immediately you will feel your thumb sink into the spinal groove. Continue to drag your thumb laterally over the transverse process until you feel it once again fall into an indentation or groove. This second groove is the costotransverse groove and you will notice that it is not as deep as the spinal groove. Practice finding the costotransverse groove because the two tests that you will learn for determining rib fixations require you to place your fingers here. Although the costotransverse groove is the best place to feel for rib fixations, it is not as useful if you are trying to palpate for torsion or subluxation.

Before you learn the two methods for determining rib fixation, let's first look at how to palpate for torsion and subluxation. Although it is

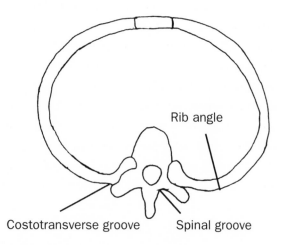

Figure 9.2

not altogether necessary, it helps if you can look at a skeleton while practicing rib palpation. The first thing to notice is that the superior borders of ribs are not as easy to feel as the inferior borders. The shape and position of these borders is such that the superior border feels less distinct than the inferior border. So don't let this feature of how the ribs are shaped mislead you into thinking you are palpating internal torsion.

To determine torsion, palpate the superior and inferior borders of the suspected rib at about the rib angle. If the rib is externally torsioned, then you will find two telltale signs: the superior border will be more prominent and the inferior less prominent than normal, and the intercostal space above the rib will be wider and the intercostal space below the rib will be narrower than normal. Internal torsion displays just the opposite features. The inferior border of the suspected rib will be more prominent and the superior border will be less prominent than normal, and the intercostal space below the rib will be wider and the intercostal space above the rib will be narrower than usual.

To determine subluxation, palpate the head of the suspected rib on the front of the rib cage at the costochondral junction and the rib angles on the posterior side of the rib cage. Then compare the suspected rib to the rib on the other side. Is the posterior rib angle of the suspected rib more anterior/posterior? Is the rib head more anterior/posterior than the rib on the other side at the costochondral junction? If the rib angle and the rib head at the costochondral junction are both more anterior in comparison to the rib on the other side, then the suspected rib is probably anteriorly subluxed. If the rib angle and the rib head at the costochondral junction are both more posterior than the rib on the other side, then the suspected rib is probably posteriorly subluxed.

Palpating ribs for torsion and subluxation can be difficult, especially on clients whose back musculature is highly developed. To increase your palpatory skills it is best for you to practice feeling these rib patterns. But fortunately, you really don't have to go through the above process of palpation to find a fixed rib and free it. You can simply put your thumb in the costotransverse groove on the suspected rib and motion test it.

Use the so-called "spring test" to motion-test ribs. Put your thumb on the suspected rib where it articulates with the costotransverse process and with firm pressure quickly push anteriorly and just as quickly release the pressure. Do this a couple of times in rapid succession so that you can feel whether the rib springs or not. If you cannot feel the rib spring, it is probably fixed. Spring test a number of ribs until you can feel the clear difference between a fixed rib that has no spring to it and a free rib that easily springs with pressure.

Another way to motion test for rib fixations is through a kind of assisted spring test. Place your client in a sitting position and ask him to put each hand on his opposite shoulder so that his arms are crossed. Stand behind your client and hold up his crossed arms at his elbows with one of your hands. Make sure that your client gives you the full weight of his arms and is not unconsciously trying to help you hold his arms up. Place your thumb in the area of the suspected rib and then smoothly but rapidly raise and lower your client's arms. As you raise his arms, push your thumb anteriorly and then let the pressure off as you lower his arms (Figures 9.3 and 9.4). If either or both the costotransverse or costovertebral joints are fixed, your thumb will not sink in an anterior direction as you raise your client's arms. If your thumb doesn't sink anteriorly as you raise your client's arms, you have discovered a fixed rib.

Both of these tests will give you all the information you need to release rib fixations, but the assisted spring test is a little more reliable and accurate, especially if you are new to palpating for rib fixations. Notice that

118

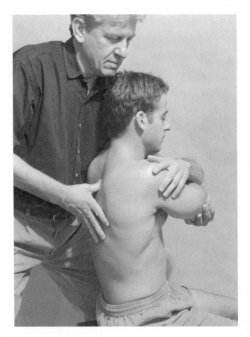

Figure 9.3

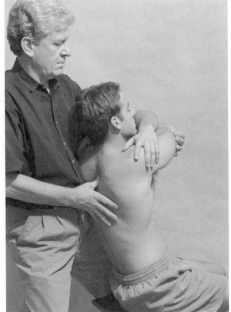

Figure 9.4

these tests only tell you which ribs are fixed but they do not also tell you whether the ribs are fixed in anterior or posterior subluxation or in external or internal torsion. Fortunately you don't really need to make these kinds of discriminations in order to use the technique for releasing ribs. You only need to know where the fixation is located.

By the way, as a method to increase evaluation skills, you should also know that rib fixations are usually accompanied by characteristic tender points in the soft tissues, illustrated in Figure 9.5, page 120. Notice that a number of these tender points are along the edge of the scapula. When clients have fixed ribs, it is quite common for them to tell you that they are experiencing pain at the edge of their scapula. However, don't be misled by where your clients tell you to look for painful spots. More often than not the pain they feel in the area of the rhomboids is secondary to and a result of the rib fixation. If you release the rhomboids and do not release the offending rib, your client's pain will return very shortly. However, after you release the rib, releasing the myofasciae along the shoulder blade will support your release of the rib.

119

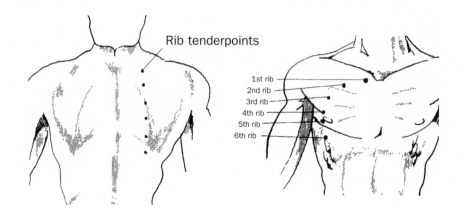

Rib tenderpoints

1st rib
2nd rib
3rd rib
4th rib
5th rib
6th rib

Figure 9.5

Another way to locate fixations is to run your thumbs or fingers down the costotransverse groove on one side of the spine and then the other, and notice if you feel something that makes you want to investigate. Do this without any preconceptions and you will be surprised by how often your fingers will land on a rib fixation. You can do the same thing in the spinal groove if you want to practice a quick way to find vertebral facet fixations. Once you gain confidence in your ability to feel for fixations in this way, you can search out dysfunctions in the same way anywhere in your client's body. This method of locating problems in your clients is quite elegant and something you can easily practice every time you treat them.

As you may remember, the first rib behaves a little differently than ribs 2–10. When the first rib becomes dysfunctional it tends to get fixed in a superior position. When it is in trouble you will also find that the scalenes will be hypertonic on the same side as the fixed rib and that there will be marked tenderness in the area of the superior aspect of the first rib near where it articulates with T1. Have you ever had the experience of doing a great job of releasing your client's cervical pain only to have him report that his neck still hurts—and that it especially hurts when he turns his head to one side where he feels the pain shooting along the right superior edge of his traps? Such a report is usually an indication that the right first rib is fixed.

There are two ways of testing for whether the first rib is in trouble. The first method is just another variation of the spring test. With your client in a sitting position, place the pad of your thumb over where the first rib articulates with T1 and spring test downwardly in a caudad direction. If it doesn't spring it is probably fixed. Another way to test the first rib is to put your client in a sitting position and place the fingers of each hand over the first ribs, with your forefingers very close to the spinal articulation and ask your client to take a deep breath. If one of the first ribs is fixed it will not move with the inhalation.

Rib Techniques

BEFORE YOU RELEASE ANY RIB FIXATIONS, BE CERTAIN THAT THE SOFT tissues of the thoracic region are adequately prepared, especially around the costotransverse, costovertebral, costochondral, and sterno-chondral regions. First release all Type II facet fixations in the thoracic spine.

All of the following techniques for releasing ribs are done with the client in a sitting position. For dysfunctions of ribs 2–10, place the finger or thumb of one hand on the costotransverse articulation and a finger of the other hand on the costochondral articulation of the dysfunctional rib (Figures 9.6, 9.7, and 9.8, pages 122–123). Slowly, but with gentle, firm pressure push your fingers toward each other. As you apply pressure, ask your client to sidebend his body to the same side as the fixed rib. Hold and wait. Follow the dance of the rib as it unwinds, releases its restrictions, and the tissue softens. Continue to hold and wait until you feel the body organize itself as much as it can around vertical and horizontal planes. You may remember from earlier chapters that there are two stages to the final release of a joint fixation. First you will feel the softening of the tissues and then, if you wait just a little longer, you may feel the orthotropic effect as your client's body organizes itself around the sagittal, transverse, and coronal planes. For most somatic practitioners feeling the body organize itself around vertical lines is the easiest. So don't worry about not feeling all of these planes come in during the release. Just practice feeling what you can and in time you will feel even more. These planes intersect at right angles and as a short hand way to talk about how the body organizes itself

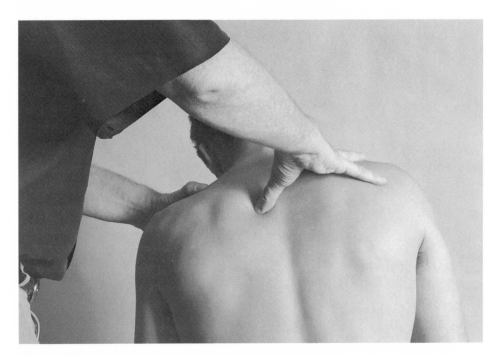

Figure 9.6

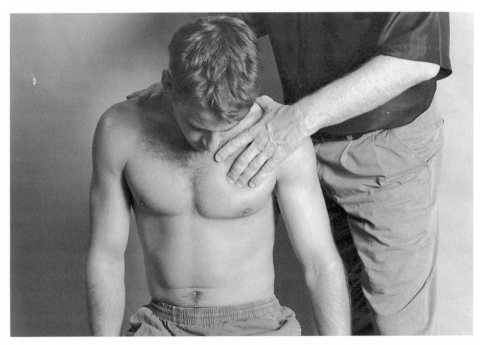

Figure 9.7

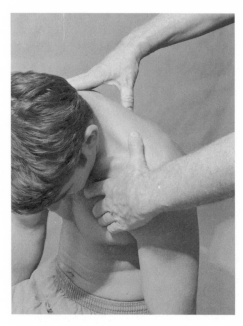

Figure 9.8

around these planes, I refer to it as orthogonal organization.

Let's suppose the rib you are attempting to release is stuck in external torsion. As the rib goes through its dance, you will notice it often moves further into external torsion before it releases. The rib will move in many odd ways, but eventually it will move further into external torsion. When the rib completes this movement it will then move out of external torsion toward a more normal position. Tracking this rib motion and taking note of its positions while you are attempting to release it is the way you determine how the rib is stuck. When the rib finally comes to rest in what is normal position in relation to the rest of the body, it will stop moving. You will then feel the tissue soften and the characteristic attempt of the body to organize orthotropically and orthogonally around the release.

For dysfunctions of the 11th and 12th ribs, place the thumb or finger of one hand as close as possible to the costovertebral articulation and the forefinger and thumb of the other hand along the length of the rib as it wraps its way around the body, as shown in Figures 9.9 and 9.10, page 124. Slowly apply gentle but firm pressure to the costovertebral junction and sidebend your client to the side on which the rib is fixed. Follow the dance and wait for the rib to release and for the body to organize orthogonally. Don't forget that there are fascial vortices in the posterior abdominal wall that are often associated with restrictions in the 11th and 12th ribs, and that these myofascial strain patterns must also be released for this technique to be fully effective.

To release these associated fascial vortices, ask your client to lie supine. If any vortices are present, they will be found medial to the tips of the 11th and 12th ribs roughly in the area of the external abdominal oblique, trans-

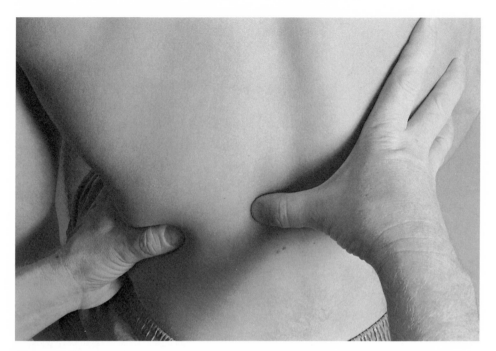

Figure 9.9

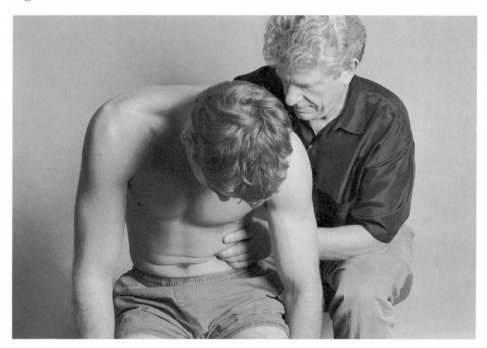

Figure 9.10

versus, and rectus abdominus. To search for these vortices, gently push the pad of your thumb or forefinger and middle finger into various places in the area just described and wait to see if your fingers are drawn down and into the tissue in a spiraling fashion, as shown in Figures 9.11, 9.12, and 9.13. If this happens you have discovered a fascial vortex. Place the forefingers, or the forefingers and middle fingers, of both hands in the area of the vortex and gently sink into the tissue waiting for the body's response. More often than not your fingers will gently follow the tissue by spiraling deeper into the vortex. When you reach the end of the spiraling, you will feel a softening of the tissue and an impulse for the vortex to unwind itself up and out of its spiral. Let this happen. Sometimes your fingers just spiral down into the tissue and the body will simply release the strain without spiraling back out. Either way the release happens, you will know the technique is finished when you feel the tissues soften and release along a vertical line. Like all releases, the body will try to organize itself orthogonally, but feeling the other planes while releasing fascial vortices is sometimes a little difficult.

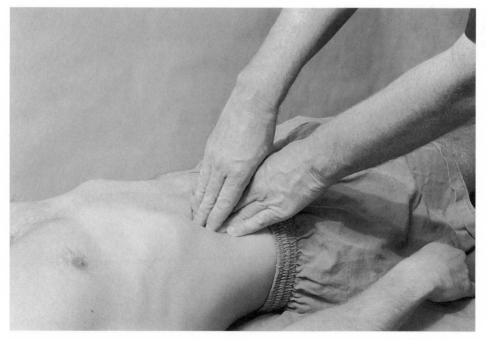

Figure 9.11

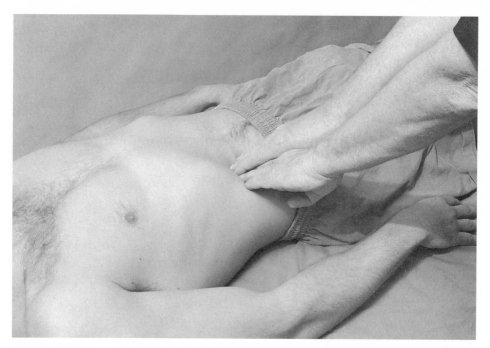

Figure 9.12

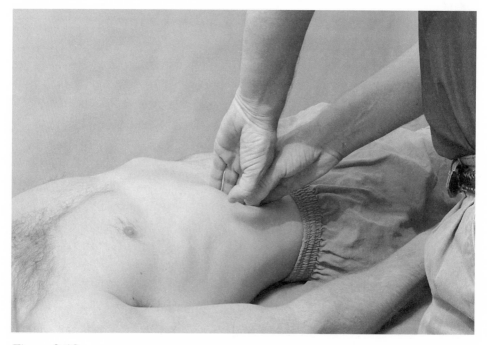

Figure 9.13

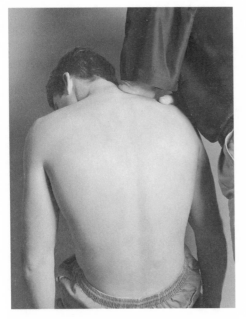

Figure 9.14

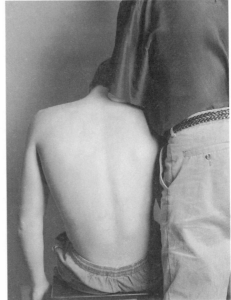

Figure 9.15

If you motion test and find a restricted first rib, more than likely it will be fixed superiorly. Let's suppose you find the restriction in the right first rib. With your client in a sitting position, snuggle the edge of your ulna (the part that is closest to your olecranon) onto your client's first rib where it attaches to T1 at the costotransverse junction. Ask your client to drop his head as far forward as is comfortable and to remain in this position while he slowly turns his head to the left. As he turns left, let your elbow sink further into the joint space (Figure 9.14). Then ask him to bring his head back to center and very slowly turn to the right, all the while keeping his head in the forward bent position (Figure 9.15). As he slowly turns right, continue to apply gentle but firm pressure in a caudad direction to the rib head. Wait for the rib to go through its unwinding, release its restriction, and for the tissues to soften. Continue with the pressure until the body organizes itself orthogonally as much as it can. Then be sure to release scalenes on the ipsilateral side.

This chapter on the ribs really brings this manual on spinal manipulation to a close. In the next and last chapter I will discuss a few odds and ends that will clarify some important points and suggest a few other techniques.

10

Odds and Ends

THE BODY IS NOT A SOFT MACHINE OR A COMPLEX THING MADE OF parts. It is a seamless unified living whole capable of adapting to an ever-changing internal and external environment. What we are tempted to call "parts" of the body are really not parts at all— our bodies are not cobbled together from pre-shaped parts the way machines are. Any attempt to take apart a body the way you might disassemble a machine into its parts only results in a heap of lifeless pieces that cannot be reassembled as a body. So we speak too loosely when we refer to the liver or brain or the foot as a part of the body. Whenever we refer to some aspect of the living body, such as the hand or the heart, we are really referring to an aspect or expression of the whole. An organ is not *in* the body in the same way a carburetor is in a car. Conceptually, we can distinguish these different aspects of the whole, but no one of these aspects is functionally separate from the whole.

What we call organs and other anatomical structures are in reality organized, unified relationships related to the living whole which is also a living, organized, unified relationship. Every unified relationship is composed of other unified relationships and every relationship is an integral aspect of other relationships. The connections, communication networks, and forces between bodily relationships are themselves unified relationships and the way they all function together is a unified relationship. What we are tempted to call parts are not only unified relationships, but also organized wholes.

These organized wholes exist in relationship to other organized wholes and overlap as networks of communication and connection that are all expressions of a deliquescent, but exquisitely and hierarchically organized whole. Some unified relationships, like the heart and brain, are more important to the survival of the whole than others. But since the body is not composed of parts, there is nothing more fundamental to the makeup and organization of the whole than the whole itself. Since the body is an irreducible complexity and not cobbled together from pre-shaped parts, every detail of the whole is an expression of the unified, seamless organization of the whole. The shape of every bone in your body, for example, is a matchless manifestation of your unique morphology.

All living organisms are self-organizing and we humans are the most highly plastic of all. Organisms persist over time because they are constantly in the process of forming and re-forming their boundaries in response to their ever-changing environments. Living beings are able to accomplish this remarkable feat in the face of persistent internal and external change because their order and organization is self-maintained and self-contained. An organism is like a fountain of water whose constituent materials are being rapidly replaced, while variations in the form remain the same over time. But unlike a fountain where the form is maintained by outside forces, organisms have the inherent power to maintain and adapt their form to their environment. Maintaining, adapting, and evolving bodily form in an ever-changing environment are part of what it means to be alive. How well our bodies accomplish these amazing feats are also an important part of what determines our level of health, happiness, and sense of well-being and freedom.

These characteristics result in a body that is also highly adaptive and plastic. If a person is injured, say in an automobile accident, her body often develops patterns of compensation in relation to the original pattern of injury. The automobile accident does not just cause a local problem with some "part" of the body, it also creates global patterns of strain that in turn affect the organization and functioning of the entire body and its relation to gravity.

The original pattern of injury more often than not is laid down on other previous injuries and postural imbalances. Along with the resulting patterns of compensation in relation to gravity, these imbalances and injury patterns result in a complicated loss of inherent plasticity and adaptability throughout the entire body. Over time, further losses in movement, plasticity, and adaptability will appear as the body struggles with gravity in its daily activities. If these complicated patterns of strain and compensation are not released, and perhaps more importantly, not released in the proper order, the body will not be able to respond properly to interventions designed to release the original injury site or any other area of dysfunction. Treating the body as an assemblage of dysfunctional parts and releasing the parts symptom by symptom is the most common way that somatic practitioners approach therapy. This methodology can be called the "corrective approach." It certainly has its place in the therapeutic arena, but it is usually less effective than the "holistic approach" which requires understanding the interconnected living whole in which all these local dysfunctions are embodied.

The human body is amazing in its interconnected, irreducible complexity and equally astounding in its seamless simplicity. The more we understand about the unified, systematic, interconnected nature of our bodies and how the whole person responds to injury *and* intervention, the better our therapy becomes. This realization means that as much as possible we must keep expanding our understanding of, and our ability to feel, this unified living whole that we are. It also means that if we want our manipulations to be long lasting, we must expand our understanding so that we can work holistically rather than just correctively. The holistic approach to somatic therapy aims not only to remediate symptoms, but also to enhance the whole person. Effective holistic somatic therapy demands that the practitioner not only be able to perceive the whole, but to also track the effects of her local manipulations on the whole.

So in a sense, even though this book is about spinal manipulation, it should also be about the whole body. But such a goal is too vast for a manual of technique. In order to make this book manageable, I have approached therapeutic intervention from the corrective perspective. Unfortunately, since the corrective approach tends to understand the client as a collection of symptoms, it is almost always just a little too shortsighted. Since so many local areas of dysfunction are tied to, and held, by more global patterns of strain, the holistic perspective is required to gain some understanding of these whole body connections. That is why I mention the holistic perspective now and also why I have taken some limited excursions into other areas of the body. Like all therapists, you want your clients to experience long-lasting relief as a result of your spinal manipulations. These digressions will help you to understand and treat some of the more significant compensations and fixations that contribute to your client's body maintaining its dysfunctions—but obviously not all of them.

The inherent difficulties with the corrective approach to therapy can only be overcome with a more complete discussion of the holistic approach. Such a discussion would have to show that the corrective approach is based on a mechanical understanding of the body that sees it as a complex thing made of parts. It would also have to articulate a proper philosophy and science of living wholes that would form the biological foundation for a holistic medical system. It would also include understanding and treating the whole body, not just the spine. Thus, we would also have to explore how to treat the cranium, the extremities, and the organs, the celomic sacs, and the many energetic dimensions, neurological and psychological dysfunctions, and so on.

Even assuming that we had all this knowledge and were able to effectively treat all these different aspects of the whole person, it would still not be enough. On what basis do we take all of the information gathered from our evaluation and prioritize all the relevant techniques into a treatment strategy that takes account of how our client's whole body can adapt to and support our interventions? How we answer the three fundamental questions of therapy is critical: What do I do first, What do I do next, and When am I finished?

After we have fully evaluated our client's kinds and levels of dysfunction, we need a way to create a treatment strategy that is based on something other than simply following already determined formulistic protocols or just treating the problems symptom by symptom. Treating clients by following a treatment recipe is a useful way to learn in the beginning stages of becoming a somatic practitioner, but this method is not fully appropriate for most clients and it is not appropriate for us as we continue to mature as therapists. In order to learn how to treat our clients in all their individuality, without the benefit of formulistic protocols, we must also know how to engage in a principle-centered clinical decision-making process. So a complete discussion of holistic somatic therapy would also require a lengthy investigation into the principles of intervention: what a principle is, how principles are different from strategies, how principles function in formulating treatment strategies, and just exactly what these principles are.

All of these important topics are obviously beyond the scope of a manual on soft-tissue techniques. But mentioning them illuminates the full scope of somatic therapy and discussing them keeps us humble by reminding us how much we have to learn.

Since we have to start somewhere, and this book marks a way to begin, let's return to a more manageable task. This chapter of the book will be devoted to a few details that I purposely left for the end. Understanding them will contribute further to your ability to manipulate the spine. Some of these details concern the issue of adaptability—in this discussion you will learn what can appropriately be called preparatory techniques. But I also want to give you a few simple ways to approach spinal curvature. You may remember that I briefly talked about curvature when I introduced what are called Type I group curves toward the end of Chapter Three. We will look at adaptability issues first and then take a brief tour of spinal curvature.

Adaptability

As I suggested above, formulating a treatment strategy that is not dependent on formulistic protocols or treating your clients symptom by symptom requires a clinical-decision making process that is based on the principles of intervention. I formulated a principle-centered decision-making process in collaboration with my colleague and friend, Jan Sultan. One of the principles is called the "Adaptability Principle." I have discussed the rationale behind this principle a number of times throughout this book. The idea behind it is simple and quite obvious: if your client's body is not capable of adapting to or accepting your intervention, then either his body will return to its dysfunctional state or your manipulation will drive strain to other areas of his body—or both. This is very often the unwelcome consequence of treating symptom by symptom. But experienced holistic therapists understand what happens when they do not properly prepare a client's body to adapt to the effects of their manipulations.

133

Your client complains that his pain returned almost immediately after your treatment, or that his pain is now worse, or has spread to other areas of his body. Of course, there could be other explanations for why this happens, but failure to prepare the client's body is certainly one of the more common reasons.

Techniques for preparing your client's body so that it can adapt to your interventions can vary from simply relaxing the appropriate tissues around a vertebra before you release its facet restriction to making sure that the body as a whole can adapt to your manipulations above and support them below. Sometimes psychological issues interfere with your intervention. It is not at all uncommon to treat clients who have been sexually and physically abused. For some of these clients every attempt you make to manipulate the pelvis and low back is met with unconscious resistance. These unfortunate clients cannot adapt to your intervention because they are not psychologically prepared to deal with the memories and emotions that might result if they were to allow changes in their bodies.

Another very important principle of intervention is the "Support Principle." It is actually a specific application of the adaptability principle and also derived from the pioneering work of Dr. Ida P. Rolf. It says that order is a function of available support in gravity. Again, the rationale behind this principle is simple and obvious: if your client's body is not able to support the changes you introduce, then either it will revert to its prior dysfunctional state or you will drive strain elsewhere—or both. If you decide to release a number of fixations in the pelvic and lumbar region, for example, and your client's legs are not under him properly supporting the pelvis and the rest of his body, then the ability of your client to hold onto the results of your treatment will be limited.

Imagine how you might proceed if your evaluation revealed that your client could neither adapt above or below, or support your interventions. You would have to create a treatment strategy that addressed all of her specific adaptability and support issues. In a situation like this, it is usually best to begin by addressing the most important adaptability issues first and the support issues last. The reason for this particular approach rests on the observation that work on the feet and legs tends to release upward through the body. If your client's body cannot adapt above to this upwardly rising wave of release that almost always results from working on feet and legs, then your manipulations could cause some nasty problems in your client's thorax, neck, and head. Only after these adaptability and support issues have been handled should you begin working to release the myofascial and joint fixations in the pelvic region.

As you probably realized, there are other principles of intervention and other considerations about how to evaluate the structural, functional, and energetic aspects of the whole person that are important to this holistic decision-making process. I mention only the support and adaptability principles because they are obvious and can be used to give you an idea of how principle-centered decision making works and a sense of how a holistic somatic practitioner operates according to principles.

In this chapter we will limit our discussion to issues of local adaptability. Discussing the more global compensations and strain patterns that manifest in a person's structural, functional, emotional, and energetic ways of being would require another book on how to evaluate these global patterns, as well as a complete discussion of the principles of intervention. To keep things simple we will only discuss those local areas of the body that are directly relevant to releasing the joint fixations we have discussed in this book.

What to Prepare

THIS SECTION DESCRIBES MANY OF THE LOCAL AREAS OF MYOFASCIAL and ligamentous dysfunction that are commonly associated with joint fixations. As a general rule, you should consider releasing these associated areas first before dealing with the specific joint fixation. You can release the tissues after you release the joint fixation, but it is usually easier on you and on your client if you release the relevant tissues first. As I mentioned previously, all the techniques I discuss in this book will work quite well if you do not attempt to release these associated soft tissue restrictions. But you definitely will be much more effective if you release these myofascial and ligamentous restrictions first. This discussion is not meant to be exhaustive, it contains only the most important areas — the ones you should always be sure not to overlook.

Also I will not devote much discussion to the techniques to use to release these areas, because there are many ways to accomplish the desired results and most readers of this book already know many of them. Besides, there are many classes and workshops on soft tissue techniques readily available to somatic practitioners in both the United States and Europe.

The most important recommendation I want to make is to find ways to release soft-tissue restrictions that do not cause unnecessary pain to your clients. When it comes to treating the human body, more is not always better. Too many soft tissue practitioners apply way too much pressure to the body and willfully push their way through the tissues. This willful application of elbows and knuckles not only causes unnecessary pain and tissue damage, it also interferes with your ability to feel the orthotropic effect. Applying the "no pain, no gain" philosophy is not the most effective approach, and can often be abusive. Use what you have learned from this book when you approach the release of myofasciae and ligaments, and don't force your way through the tissue. Let your client's body tell you what it wants and how it wants to release. If you respect the way the body wants to release and find its way to its own inherent order, you can apply heavy pressure and not worry about causing unnecessary pain. Sink into the tissue and wait for the dance. Your clients will be much happier if you do and your results will also be better.

Dr. Rolf, the creator and founder of Rolfing, taught a shotgun technique that is sometimes useful for releasing the musculature of the back, but it also has its dangers. Since this technique has gained a lot of popularity among many other somatic practitioners, I want to make sure you know when to use it and when not to.

The technique works this way: place your client in a sitting position and lean your right elbow on his right upper back at about the cervicothoracic junction over the spinal groove and transverse processes. Don't use the point of your elbow, use the flatter aspect just superior to the olecranon. Let your elbow sink into the tissue by letting your weight do most of the work. Ask your client to slowly bend forward (Figure 10.1). As he does so, keep your pressure up and slide your elbow down his back at a rate that keeps up with the rate at which the tissue releases. Be sure to slide your elbow all the way down and through the tissue around the sacroiliac joint (Figure 10.2). Ask your client to sit up and repeat the process on the left side. You can run your elbow down your client's back a couple of times on each side. As a matter of course you may even release some closed

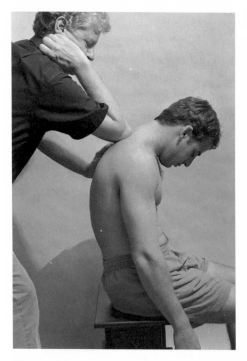 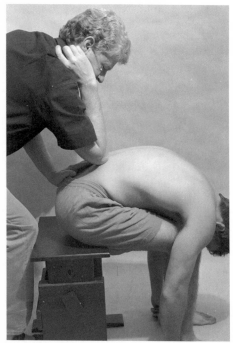

Figure 10.1 *Figure 10.2*

fixed facets. But as you also probably realized, this technique will have no effect on all the open-fixed facets.

This technique is a very useful shotgun approach for releasing the back musculature. But be careful with it. If your client has severe back pain, degenerative joint disease, and/or disc problems, don't use this technique, because you can actually make her back pain much much worse. If your client has disc problems you may even cause the disc to herniate further.

Any time you release sacroiliac, iliosacral, or lumbar facet fixations, check the hamstrings, the gluteals, the pelvic rotators, the adductors, the quadratus lumborum, the psoas, the myofasciae of the lumbar and thoracolumbar regions, and the pelvic ligaments. Normalize those areas where you find strain, tightness, and imbalances from side to side. Figure 10.3, page 138, shows the complex ligamentous structure of this area. When releasing the sacrum, be sure to pay special attention to the sacrotuberous (7), sacrospinous (6), sacroiliac (5), and the piriformis (Figure 10.4). When you are releasing the sacrum, L5, and L4 also be certain you check

137

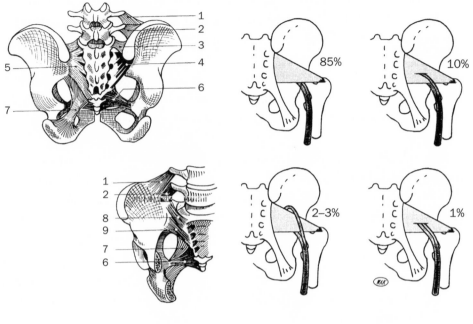

Figure 10.3   *Figure 10.4*

the iliolumbar ligaments (1 and 2).

If your client is complaining of sciatic pain, you want to be sure to evaluate L4, L5, the sacrum, the ligaments previously mentioned, and especially the piriformis muscle. It is usually not enough to release the compression on the sciatic nerve at L4 on L5, because L5, the sacrum, the ligaments, and the pelvic rotators, especially the piriformis, are often part of the problem. The drawings in Figure 10.4 present four different ways the sciatic nerve can thread its way around or through the piriformis and the percentage of time each shows up in the human population. It also dramatically illustrates why sciatic pain can be maintained by a dysfunctional piriformis muscle long after the compression on the nerve root has been alleviated. So always check the piriformis muscle when you are releasing the sacrum or dealing with sciatic pain.

The hamstrings almost always contribute to maintaining strain and fixation through the lumbar and pelvic regions. Time and again I have watched a sacrum derotate as I released the hamstrings. When you see lumbar sidebending, more than likely you will also see both a tight and short psoas and quadratus lumborum on the side to which the spine is sidebending. Think of the lumbar spine as a tent pole and the psoas muscles as guy wires. Every lumbar vertebrae is attached to the psoas and if one of these guy wires is pulling more than the other it is sure to unbalance the spine. Even if you just find the common dysfunctional pattern where L4 and L5 are sidebent and rotated to the same side, you should treat the psoas and the quadratus lumborum on the side to which L4 and L5 are sidebent.

You should also pay attention to the adductors, especially where they attach at the pelvic ramus. Manipulating dysfunctionally shortened adductors will greatly contribute to your attempt to release the sacrum and lumbars. Since the adductors and the psoas are intimately connected in this area, if you release the adductors you should also release the psoas. And then make sure that the lumbar and thoracolumbar myofasciae will permit the full release of this area. It is very common to find myofascial strain and tightness in the thoracolumbar region of clients who have had a history of low back pain.

Even if you have prepared all the associated tissues properly, and done a great job of releasing all the fixations in the sacrum, lumbars, and pelvis, sometimes your client complains that he still has just a little bit of pain and stiffness either in the center of his sacrum or around the SI joints and ILA's. If this happens, you probably need to be more specific in how you release the associated myofasciae and ligaments. Ask your client to sit on your treatment bench and forward bend as far over as he is comfortable. Use the knuckles of both hands to apply 20 to 30 pounds of pressure to the area around the right side of the lumbosacral junction. Sink into the tissues and wait for them to respond (Figure 10.5, page 140). When you feel the tissues begin to soften, slide inferiorly along the right SI joint with your left knuckle on the medial side of the SI joint and the right knuckle on the lateral side of the SI joint. Slide through this area at a speed that matches tissues' release, then do the other side. If your client is complaining of lingering pain in the center of the sacrum, place the knuckles of each hand close together, apply the same amount of pressure starting at the lumbosacral junction, sink into the tissues, wait for them to soften, and slide inferiorly along the body of the sacrum. This technique can be somewhat intense for the client (meaning it may hurt), but it is very

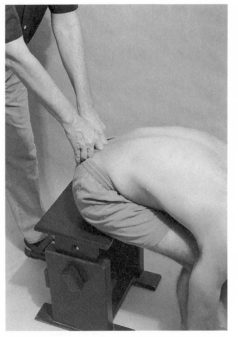

Figure 10.5

effective for releasing this last bit of strain. Apply the technique a couple of times in a way that your client can tolerate and he should feel immediate relief.

Whenever you release fixations at one end of the spine, be sure you attend to the other end and release whatever fixations you find. A change in the lumbars can create change in the cervicals and visa versa. So it is always a good idea to make sure that both ends of the spine are happy and free before you send your clients home.

Before you release facet restrictions in the neck, use whatever techniques you know to ease and release the muscles and fascial sheets along the back and sides of the neck and the tissues around the OA. Figure 10.6 shows a useful shotgun technique you may want to try. Pick up your client's head and rest the back of his head in the crook of your right hand (the part formed by webbing of your thumb and forefinger). With the index and/or middle fingers of your left hand, apply pressure and sink into the tissue of the left spinal groove around the atlas. When you feel the tissue soften, slide inferiorly with the fingers of your right hand to about T1 and T2. Reverse your hands and treat the right cervical spinal groove the same way. Besides releasing the posterior myofasciae, this technique will often release some of the less severe fixed-closed facets. Of course it won't release the fixed-open facets, but because it does double-duty in releasing soft tissues and extension restrictions, it saves you time and energy.

Whenever you work in the neck area be sure that you always attend to the suboccipital muscles. This region is almost always involved with dysfunctional patterns in the neck. In Figure 10.7, notice how all of these suboccipital muscles, with the exception of the obliquus capitus inferior (3) (and the interspinous muscles), attach to the base of the occiput. The

140

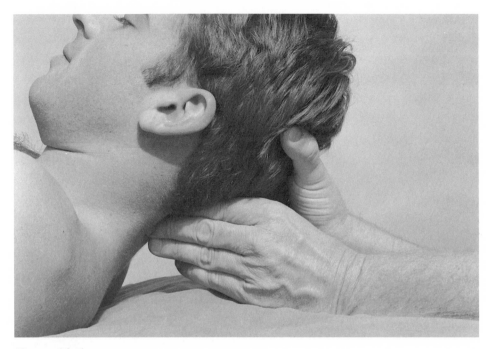

Figure 10.6

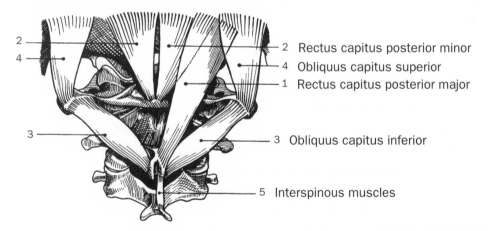

Figure 10.7

rectus capitus posterior major (1) attaches to the spinous process of C2 and the occiput, the rectus capitus posterior minor (2) attaches to C1 and the occiput, the obliquus capitus superior (4) attaches to the transverse

141

process of C1 and the occiput, and the obliquus capitus inferior (3) attaches to C2 and the transverse process of C1. New dissection procedures have revealed the existence of a previously unknown muscle and ligament complex that extends from the suboccipital muscles to the dura mater that surrounds the brain. When you put this newly understood connection to the cranial dura together with what happens when the suboccipital muscles get tight and short in response to stress or facet restrictions, then you easily understand why these muscles can be the source of a real pain in the neck—and some really nasty headaches. So always make sure this entire region is soft and at ease before you end your treatment.

Before you release ribs, it is very helpful to ease the back musculature and the tissues along the sides and the front of the rib cage, especially around the sternum, and the costochondral and ster-nochondral junctions. Pay special attention to the inter-costal muscles, especially above and below the fixed ribs you plan to treat, and make sure they are at ease. As I mentioned in Chapter Nine, the rhomboids are always involved in rib restrictions, but you should also pay attention to the levator scapulae and serratus posterior superior muscles.

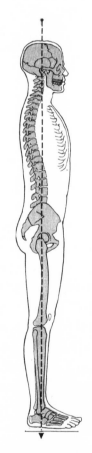

Curvature

Treating curvatures in the human body is a very complicated affair. Curvature is inherent to our bodies and along with curvature comes asymmetry. Many schools of manual and movement therapy look upon all bodily curvature and asymmetry as dysfunctional and try their best to intervene and change these patterns. Many of these schools adhere to some notion of an "Ideal Body" that they use as a standard against which to evaluate their clients' bodies.

A good example of the theory of the ideally aligned body and its use in evaluating dysfunction is described by Kendall and McCreary.[1] Pictured in Figure 10.8, the ideal body is defined by dropping a plumb line through the

Figure 10.8

center of gravity of the body (i.e., slightly anterior to the first or second sacral segment). If the centers of gravity of the other segments fall along this plumb line, it is considered properly aligned. According to this view, the line of gravity should fall through the middle of the ear lobe, through the middle of the acromion process, through the greater trochanter, slightly anterior to the axis of the knee joint, and slightly anterior to the lateral malleolus. This concept of the ideal body has influenced many practitioners, who often inappropriately evaluate and treat their patients in terms of how well they measure up to this external ideal. Unfortunately this conception rests on the gratuitous assumption that the human body is equally dense throughout. Since it is not, it cannot be lined up the way you might align a pile of blocks.

Like Dr. Rolf and many other theorists, Kendall and McCreary assume that the closer bodies match this ideal, the better they function. This view has some truth to it, but when applied indiscriminately to every patient, dysfunction can result. Consider a few obvious examples. A pregnant woman or an overweight patient with a large "pot belly" would be aligned in a most peculiar way if any attempt were made to balance them around the line of gravity. Consider patients with upper neuron problems like cerebral palsy. In many of these patients, any attempt to align their heads on top of their bodies, as this ideal recommends, will often result in tonal overflow to the extremities, possible increase in non-functional reflex patterns of movement, and loss of control.

We shouldn't automatically assume that clients are manifesting some sort of dysfunction solely because their bodies do not measure up to this external ideal of good posture. Any attempt to completely rid the body of curvature and asymmetry is a hopeless enterprise. If such an impossible goal could be realized, it would probably cause the utmost distress and pain to the poor person who received this well-intentioned therapy.

As you might well imagine, most theorists who believe that there is standard that all bodies should measure up to also believe in an "Ideal Spine." Figure 10.9, page 144, shows Dr. Rolf's view of what this ideal spine should look like. But when you compare her view to what actually exists, you see there is quite a disparity. The form and curvature of any given spine is a unique expression of the morphology and functioning of the entire body. If you look carefully at the great differences between your clients' spines,

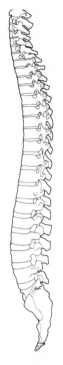

you will realize that any attempt to manipulate them to match the shape of the ideal spine is an impossible goal. Do you remember Figure 10.10? It accompanied the discussion of the shape of the facets of the innominate and sacrum in Chapter Seven. Notice how clearly it shows the relationship between the facets and the shape of the sacrum. The impossibility of ever manipulating the sacrum of spine A in Figure 10.10 toward a position like spine B's is all too obvious. There is no way to change the position of a sacrum with that shape, because the shape of the facets would never permit it. Remember, the shape of any given bone is an expression of the unique morphology of the entire body. If you cannot get the sacrum into this idealized position, you will never get the spine there either. I have seen too many dysfunctional spines that look just like the ideal spine and many very functional spines look like spine A. So we cannot automatically conclude that

Figure 10.9

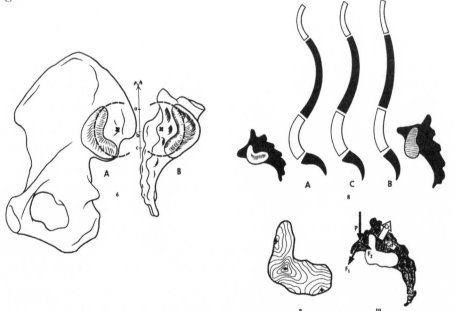

Figure 10.10

144

just because a client's spine or body doesn't measure up to an ideal that it is dysfunctional and in need of manipulation. In fact, many times the attempt to make a client's body conform to an ideal either has no effect or, worse, actually creates further dysfunction.

Somatic practitioners in every discipline have been taught to evaluate clients by comparing their bodies to some conscious or unconscious somatic ideal. Too often, contour, position, curvature, and asymmetry are used as the only indicators of somatic dysfunction and disorder. Once we see through the limitations of evaluating our clients against these somatic ideals, we will see the odd contours and the odd positioning of segments, curvatures, and asymmetries that show up in every body in an entirely different light. All of these odd patterns must be evaluated in terms of the unique limitations and possibilities for each body and each body type. Rejecting the notions of an ideal body and ideal positions for individual segments does not undermine our ability to evaluate our clients' bodies. There are recognizable patterns of dysfunction that show up in every body type, as well as common patterns of asymmetry that show up in various types of bodies, and there are asymmetries unique to the individual client. Some of these patterns are associated with dysfunction and some are not. When patterns that are associated with structural, functional, and energetic fixations are properly managed in accordance with individual needs, overall function can be restored and enhanced.

So when you see oddly positioned segments, curvature, and asymmetries, what do you do about them? My suggestion is that you view an oddly positioned segment or curvature as no more than a clue to possible somatic dysfunction or disorder, not the certainty of it. So always look for loss of function in the form of fixations first (myofascial, articular, energetic, etc). Unless accompanied by some level of fixation, asymmetries and curvatures may not be even clinically significant. Asymmetries, oddly positioned segments, curvatures, and odd contours do not always demand intervention. When they do demand attention and manipulation, it is usually under the following conditions: 1) when they are accompanied by a fixation or fixations (at the structural, functional, and/or energetic levels), 2) when they contribute to a dysfunction or fixation, or 3) when manipulating them will clearly enhance the overall functioning of the whole.

So our job is to always try to understand and recognize the common patterns of dysfunction without losing sight of the uniqueness of each individual client and how her organism is organized as a whole. For each individual, the appropriate position of structures is determined by appropriate function. If a segment seems to be in an odd position, but works the way it is supposed to, don't mess with it. The same is true for all local and global asymmetries. A perceived asymmetry may be dysfunctional in one body and entirely functional and normal in another. Appropriate function is determined by understanding what is possible in relation to each individual's unique patterns of changing and unchanging limitations. In turn, these limitations must be seen in terms of how well the person has adapted to gravity and his or her environment. Position can never be abstracted from what is functionally appropriate for each individual in relation to gravity and the environment.

So what is normal, then? Etymologically, "normal" is rooted in the idea of measuring up to a norm, model, or pattern, like a carpenter's square. This meaning is the one most often associated with somatic idealism. But "normal" also carries another meaning. It can mean "natural" in the sense of "being in accordance with the inherent nature of a person or a thing." This meaning is at work when we say that a person is a natural-born artist or healer.

When I use the word "normal" I mean it in this second sense as being natural or inherent to the being of the whole person. This concept of "normal" is clearly quite different in scope and implication from the idea of measuring up to a norm, statistical average, or standard that is external to the body. Templates and norms make sense when your aim is to mass produce machines and other non-living products. Templates and norms are important in the development of quality controls. But our bodies are not machines or products, and it makes little sense to claim that all human bodies function best when they measure up to some external standard or statistical average.

"Normal" in the sense in which I use it, refers to what is appropriate and optimal for each individual person. It cannot be determined without a careful case-by-case examination of what is possible for each person, given the fixations and limitations inherent to his or her body. Normal is also not a static state that we can attain permanently. Living organisms are self-organizing, self-regulating wholes characterized by the continual ongoing attempt to balance, organize, enhance, and harmonize their lives. Given the tremendous plasticity and resulting diversity that actually exist among humans, clearly there cannot be one ideal way for every body or every segment of the body. Our world and lives are always in flux, and, whether our bodies maintain severe fixations or not, we are always striving toward becoming more fully ourselves. Some of our limitations are time-bound and changeable and some are not. What is not changeable in the present may be changeable in the future. What is changeable for one person may not be for another. Normality is an achievement that is won again and again in the course of our lives.

As a somatic therapist you are always up against three limitations: your own limitations as a therapist, the limitations of the therapeutic discipline that you learned, and the limitations of your client. Some of these limitations cannot be overcome. Most forms of manual therapy will not cure cancer, for example. But many of these limitations can be overcome. For instance, you can always learn more and improve your skills. What often appear to be severe limitations in your clients can change over time and what was incapable of changing yesterday may change tomorrow. So we must learn to recognize and respect what we can change today, what we can change in the future, and what we cannot change at all—and of course, how to tell the difference. As somatic therapists our goal is not to make clients measure up to some external standard that we impose on them by means of somatic ideals and formulistic protocols, but to try to discover the limitations that stand in the way of them becoming who they are and then to release their fixations in the right order. Normality is not a matter of measuring up to an ideal form or way of functioning, but a matter of uncovering what is natural or inherent in the being of the whole. Somatic therapy is, therefore, best practiced as a process of discovery, not as an act of imposing predetermined standards on our clients by means of formulistic protocols.

Let's return to the more practical issues at hand and look at how to deal with curvature. As I mentioned earlier, curvature is a complicated affair. As you know, the spine has a number of curves in the anterior/posterior dimension. These are the lumbar lordosis, the thoracic kyphosis, and the cervical lordosis. These A/P curves can be shallow or deep, depending on the structure of each person. And like all curvature, understanding them

requires understanding the structure of the whole body.

We are not going to discuss how
to manipulate these A/P curves, but
rather only Type I curves where
there is an appreciable lateral devi-
ation from the sagittal axis. The drawing in Figure 10.11 is a schematic
representation of a scoliosis that displays how sidebending and rotation
are coupled to opposite sides. There
are four places in the spine where
the curve might cross over and bend
in the opposite direction. These typical transition points are the lumbosacral, the thoracolumbar, the
cervicothoracic, and atlantocciptal

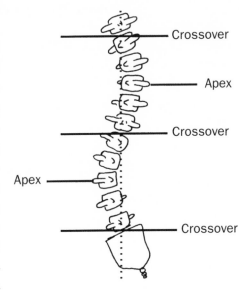

Figure 10.11

junctions. Three of these transitional junctions are displayed schemati-
cally in the drawing. You can almost always count on these crossover points
being the site of myofascial strain and tightness. There are many different kinds of laterally deviated curvatures and no two are the same. But
they all involve complicated twisting patterns that go through the entire
body from the cranium to the feet and they all involve varying degrees of
characteristic changes in the shape of the bones. Figure 10.12 shows the
direction of the scoliosis and its effect on the shape of a vertebra. Notice,
for example, how the shape of the facets and the spinal canal have been
modified by the twisting forces of the curvature. Since the shape of the
vertebrae and other bones of the body sometimes have been so profoundly
modified by the scoliosis, your ability to affect curvature will be constrained
by these bony changes.

You should always remember that a scoliosis is really a curvature that
twists and spirals throughout the whole body at every level—it is not just
a curvature of the spine. Any attempt to manipulate the spine without
addressing how the entire body is involved in the curvature is almost always
hopeless. Before you can expect any significant and lasting change, you
must make sure the cranium, the pelvis, the extremities, and the ribs are

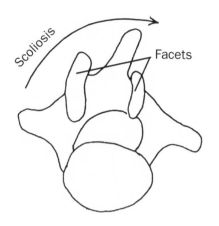

Figure 10.12

able to adapt to any unwinding of the curvature you might manage. Many times a curvature will wind its way down more into one leg than the other and releasing the compensatory patterns in that leg can sometimes significantly change the curvature.

Treating a scoliosis requires being able to perceive the whole with all its compensatory patterns and being able to track the effect of your manipulations on the whole. This is a big and complicated job. A scoliosis is a multidimensional shape that does not respond to a two-dimensional treatment approach. If you had a magic wand that permitted you to only affect the spine by forcing the S-shaped curvature straight (the way that surgically implanting Harrington rods does, for example), you would alter the sidebending without significantly changing the rotational force and, as a result, send a mess of spirals and compensatory strain patterns throughout the entire body. The holistic approach is really the best method for treating a scoliosis, because it is based on seeing and treating the whole. The corrective approach is almost always less than satisfactory. A holistic approach sometimes produces amazing results, especially when the curvature is not too pronounced and has not dramatically spun its way down into the legs or up into the cranium. In some clients you may see an actual lessening of the curve and in other cases no significant change at all. What you can reasonably hope for is a general lengthening of the body and the spine, and greater freedom and mobility throughout your client's body. Lengthening the body and the spine gives the scoliosis a softer and less compressed appearance.

Technique for Type I Group Curvatures

THE TECHNIQUE FOR TREATING TYPE I CURVATURES WAS CREATED BY MY colleague, Jim Asher, an advanced Rolfing Instructor. If you keep all the above considerations in mind, you may find his approach very useful.

You can certainly attempt to apply the technique without addressing the whole body, provided you make sure both ends of the spine are relatively free and at ease, that you have released iliosacral, sacroiliac, and all spinal facet (including the OA) and rib restrictions. If you release these areas first, you will not cause any harm to your client if you do not address the rest of the body—you may even see some surprising results.

Some group curvatures are easy to see and others are quite difficult. If you are not quite sure which way the spine is sidebent, ask you client to stand or sit and sidebend to the right and then to the left. If your client can sidebend more easily to the right than the left, you will notice that in right sidebending the curve is clear and pronounced while in left sidebending the spinal curvature is not as pronounced. You will also notice that in right sidebending the vertebrae will rotate more than they do in left sidebending. Check each curve in the spine the same way and note where the apex of each curve is on the convex side.

In preparation for understanding this technique, also notice how on the convex side of the curve the errectors are pulled toward, and packed in close to, the spine in a way that seems to diminish the depth of the spinal groove. On the concave side the errectors are pulled away from the spine and seem to be lying flat across the ribs.

Let's assume your client has a curvature like the one previously illustrated. His lumbar spine is right sidebent and left rotated and his thoracic spine is left sidebent and right rotated. For ease of understanding we will start on the thoracic spine. Place your client in a side-lying position on his left side with his left arm behind him, as shown in Figure 10.13. This position challenges the existing sidebending and rotational pattern. Place your fingers (Figure 10.14), elbow (Figure 10.15, page 152), or knuckles in the right spinal groove along the convexity of the curvature. Sink into the spinal groove, wait for the tissues to soften, and then push in a lateral direction away from the spine. Your effort should be partly directed toward freeing the tissue from being packed in too close to the spinal groove. If you start at the bottom of the convexity, push laterally as you move superiorly. If you start at the top of the convexity, push laterally as you move inferiorly. Be sure to put some extra effort into the apex of the curve.

Then ask your client to roll over onto his other side. But don't ask him to lay with his arm behind his back. Place your elbow (Figure 10.16),

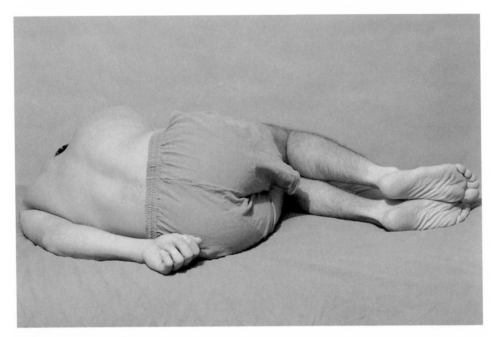

Figure 10.13

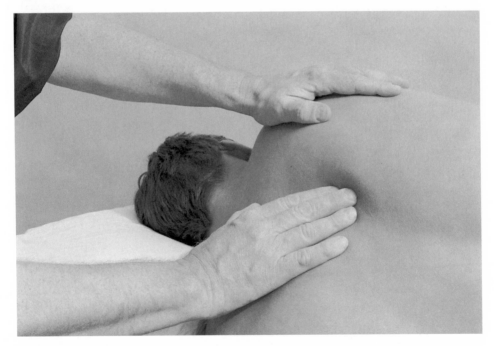

Figure 10.14

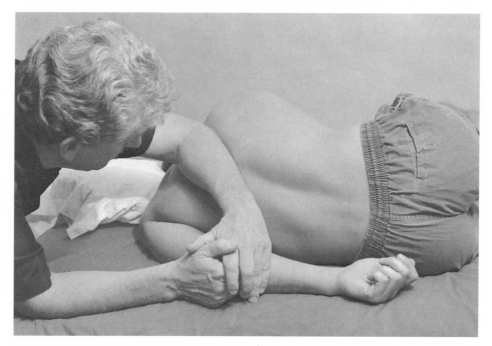

Figure 10.15

fingers, or knuckles (Figure 10.17) on the lateral borders of the erectors along the concavity of the curvature. Sink into the tissue as if you were trying to get under the erectors, wait for the softening, and then push in a medial direction toward the spine. Since these tissues are pulled wide and away from the spine, your effort is directed at easing them toward the spine.

The technique for treating the lumbar curvature is exactly the same. The only difference is how you position your client's legs to challenge his right sidebending, left rotational pattern. Use the side-lying position again and instruct your client to lay on his right side with his right knee slightly bent. In order to challenge the curvature a bit more, ask him to place his left leg in front of his body and bend his knee to 90 degrees as shown in Figure 10.18, page 154. Work in the left spinal groove along the length of the convexity of the curvature. Again, apply pressure laterally, as if you were trying to release the tissues away from the spinal groove and put a little more effort into the apex of the curve (Figure 10.19). Turn your client over on his left side, but this time make sure he keeps his knees

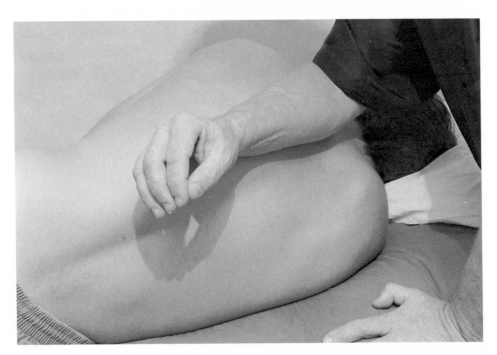

Figure 10.16

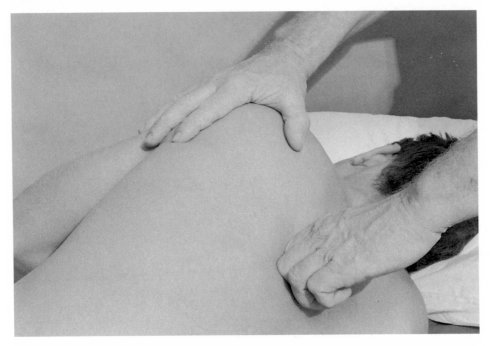

Figure 10.17

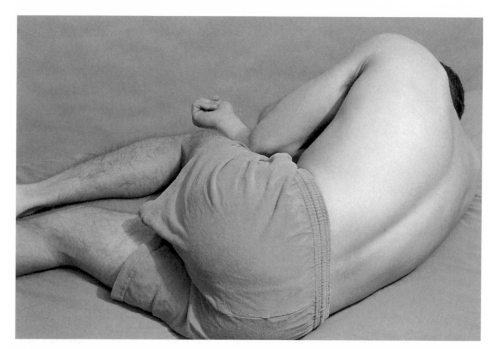

Figure 10.18

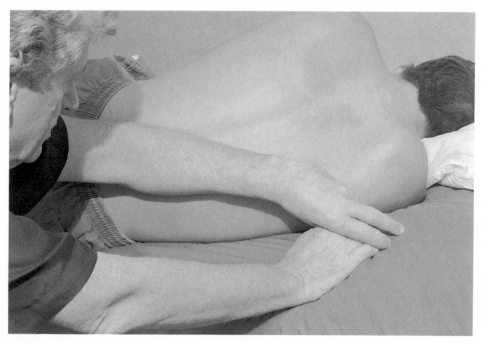

Figure 10.19

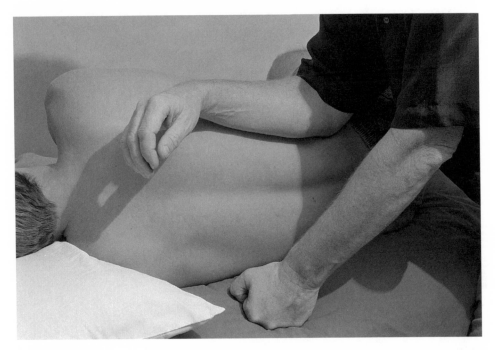

Figure 10.20

together and slightly bent. Apply pressure to the lateral borders of the errectors toward the spine along the length of the concavity of the curve (Figure 10.20).

Experiment with this technique, because on occasion it may produce surprising results. Sometimes you will see an actual reduction or lengthening of the curvature. Many times you will see a general improvement in range of motion throughout the entire spine, but sometimes you will see no obvious change at all. Always try to see the whole person with whom you are working and track the effects of your local manipulations on the whole, making sure your client can adapt to your interventions.

Remember that this book is just an introduction to the spine and I have left out some discussion of the odd things spines do. For example, the cervical vertebrae have a bad habit of side slipping in some clients. Also, many people's spines have vertebrae that have slipped just a little bit too posterior. They are not full blown examples of what is called a retrolisthesis, but they are just posterior enough to cause some loss of motion through the entire spine. I have also discovered that the facets can be fixed in planes other than the ones presented in this book. Unfortunately, delineating the tests and techniques for addressing these fixations would make this book unnecessarily complicated. As you probably suspected, not everybody is in full agreement that the spine works in the ways this book describes. This is no surprise, but if you use the information and techniques presented here, they will serve you well. Above all else, don't forget to do everything you can to improve your understanding, your technical skills, and your ability to see and feel your way into the simple complexity of what we humans truly are in relation to all of *this* to which we are neither identical nor separate.

Good luck! It has been a pleasure writing this book for you.

Note

1. Kendall, Florence Peterson and McCreary, Elizabeth Kendall. *Muscles: Testing and Function.* Third edition, Baltimore: (Williams and Wilkins), 1983.

BIBLIOGRAPHY

Basmajian, John V. and Rich Nyberg, editors. *Rational Manual Therapies,* Baltimore: Williams and Wilkins, 1993.

Bond, Mary. *Balancing your Body: A Self-Help Approach to Rolfing Movement,* Rochester, Vermont: Healing Arts Press, 1993.

Bortoft, Henri. *The Wholeness of Nature: Goethe's Way toward a Science of Conscious Participation in Nature,* Hudson, New York: Lindisfarne Press, 1996.

Cailliet, Rene. *Low Back Syndrome, Edition 4.* Philadelphia, Pennsylvania: F.A. Davis Company, 1988.

Scoliosis: Diagnosis and Management, Philadelphia: F.A. Davis Company, 1975.

Churchland, Patricia Smith. *Neurophilosophy: Toward a Unified Science of the Mind/Brain,* Cambridge, Massachusetts: The MIT press,1990.

Cottingham, John T. "Effect of Soft Tissue Mobilization on Pelvic Inclination Angle, Lumbar Lordosis, and Parasympathtic Tone: Implications for Treatment of Disabilities Associated with Lumbar Degenerative Joint Disease." Paper presented on March 19, 1992, to the National Center of Medical Rehabilitation Research of the National Institute of Child Health and Human Development, Bethesda, Maryland. Reprinted in *Rolf Lines,* Spring,1992, pp 42–45.

_____. *Healing Through Touch: A History and Review of the Physiological Evidence.* Boulder, Colorado: Rolf Institute, 1985.

_____. with Jeffrey Maitland. "Integrating Manual and Movement Therapy with Philosophical Counseling for Treatment of a Patient with Amyotrophic Lateral Sclerosis: A Case Study that Explores the Principles of Holistic Intervention," in *Alternative Therapies in Health and Medicine,* Vol. 6, No. 2, 2000, p. 128, pp. 120–127.

_____. with Steven W. Porges and K. Richmond. "Shifts in Pelvic Inclination Angle and Parasympathic Tone Produced By Rolfing Soft Tissue

Manipulation," in *Physical Therapy* Vol.68, 1988, pp. 1364–1370.

_____. with Steven W. Porges and T. Lyon. "Soft Tissue Mobilization (Rolfing pelvic lift) and Associated Changes in Parasympathetic Tone in Two Age Groups," in *Physical Therapy,* Vol. 68, 1988, pp.352–356.

_____. with Jeffrey Maitland. "A Three-Paradigm Treatment Model Using Soft Tissue Mobilization and Guided Movement-Awareness Techniques for a Patient with Chronic Low Back Pain: A Case Study," in *Journal of Orthopedic Sports Physical Therapy,* Vol. 26, No. 3, 1997, pp. 155–167.

DiGiovanna, Eileen L. and Stanley Schiowitz, editors. *An Osteopathic Approach to Diagnosis and Treatment,* Philadelphia, Pennsylvania: J.B. Lippencott Company, 1991.

Flury, Hans. *Die Neue Leichtigkeit des Körpers: Grundlagen der normalen Bewegung Übungen und Selbsthilfe für Alltag und Freizeit,* München: Deutscher Taschenbuch Verlag, 1995.

_____. *Notes on Structural Integration,* a journal series on Structural Integration from 1986 to the present. Published in Switzerland but also available from the Rolf Institute.

Greenman, Phillip E. *Principles of Manual Medicine, second edition,* Baltimore, Maryland: Williams and Wilkins, 1996.

Hammer, Warren I. *Functional Soft Tissue Examination and Treatment by Manual Methods,* Gaithersburg, Maryland: Aspen Publishers, 1991.

Kapandji, I.A. *The Physiology of the Joints, Volumes 1, 2,and 3,* New York, New York: Churchill Livingstone, 1974.

Kendall, Florence Peterson and Elizabeth Kendall McCreary. *Muscles: Testing and Function, third edition,* Baltimore, Maryland: Williams and Wilkins, 1983.

Langebartel, David A., illustrated by Robert H. Ulrich, Jr. *The Anatomical Primer: An Embryological Explanation of Human Gross Morphology,* Baltimore: University Park Press, 1977.

Maitland, Jeffrey. "An Ontology of Appreciation: Kant's Aesthetics and the Problem of Metaphysics," *Journal of the British Society for Phenomenology,* Vol. 13, No. 1, January 1982, pp. 45–68.

_____. A Phenomenology of Fascia, "in *Somatics,* Vol. III, No. 1, Autumn 1980, pp. 15–21.

_____. "Creative Performance: The Art of Life," in *Research in Phenomenology,* Vol. X, 1980, pp. 278–303.

_____. "Creativity," in *The Journal of Aesthetics and Art Criticism*, Vol. XXXIV, No. 4, Summer, 1976, pp. 397–409.

_____. "Das Boot," in *Rolf Lines*, Rolf Institute, June 1993, pp. 1–7.

_____. "The Palintonic Lines of Rolfing," *Rolf Lines*, Rolf Institute, January\February 1991, p.1, pp.43–49.

_____. "Perception and the Cognitive Theory of Life: or How Did Matter Become Conscious of Itself?" in *Rolf Lines*, Rolf Institute, Vol. XXVII, No. 4, Fall 1999, pp. 5–13.

_____. "Radical Somatics and Philosophical Counseling," invited paper presented at the Annual Meetings of the Eastern Division of the American Philosophical Association, December 28, 1998. Also in *Rolf Lines*, Rolf Institute, Vol.XXVII, No. 2, Spring 1999, pp. 29–40.

_____. "Rolfing as a Third Paradigm Approach," in *Rolf Lines*, Rolf Institute, Spring 1992, pp. 46–49.

_____. *Spacious Body: Explorations in Somatic Ontology*. Berkeley, California: North Atlantic Books, 1995.

_____. "What is Metaphysics?" in *Rolf Lines*, Rolf Institute, July/August 1990, pp. 6–9.

_____. "What is the Recipe ?" in *Rolf Lines*, Rolf Institute, June/July 1991, pp.1–4.

_____. with Jan Sultan, "Definition and Principles of Rolfing," *Rolf Lines*, Rolf Institute, Spring 1992, pp.16–20.

Mennell, John Mcm. *Back Pain*, Boston: Little, Brown, and Company, 1960.

_____. Joint Pain, Boston: Little, Brown, and Company, 1964.

Olhgren, Gael, and David Clark. "Natural Walking," *Rolf Lines*, Rolf Institute, 995, pp. 21–29.

Oschman, James L. 'The Connective Tissue and Myofascial Systems," paper published by the Aspen Research Institute, Boulder, Colorado, 1981, available through the Rolf Institute.

_____. Readings on the Scientific Basis of Bodywork. Dover, NH: N.O.R.A.; 1997.

_____. "The Structure and Properties of Ground Substances, "in *American Zoologist*, Vol. 24, No.1, 1984, pp. 199–215.

Northrup, George W, editor. *The Physiological Basis of Osteopathic Medicine*, New York, New York: The Postgraduate Institute of Osteopathic Medicine and Surgery, 1970

Rolf, Ida P. *Ida Rolf Talks About Rolfing and Physical Reality.* Edited by Rose-mary Feitis. New York, New York: Harper and Row, 1978.

_____. Rolfing: The Integration of Human Structures. New York, New York: Harper and Row, 1977.

Rose, Steven. *Lifelines: Biology, Freedom, Determinism,* London: Penguin Books, 1997.

Schultz, Louis R. and Rosemary Feitis. *The Endless Web: Fascial Anatomy and Physical Reality,* Berkeley: North Atlantic Books, 1996.

Schwind, Peter. *Alles in Lot: Korperliches and Seelisches Gleichwicht durch Rolfing.* München: Goldman Verlag, 1985.

Shafer, R.C. with L. J. Faye. *Motion Palpation and Chiropractic Technique—Principles of Dynamic Chiropractic,* Huntington Beach, California: The Motion Palpation Institute, 1989.

Steiner, Rudolf. *Goethean Science,* Spring Valley, New York: Mercury Press, 1988.

Sultan, Jan H. "Toward a Structural Logic," in *Notes on Structural Integration,* Published and edited by Hans Flury, 1986, pp. 12–16. Available from the Rolf Institute.

Ward, Robert C., executive editor. *Foundations for Osteopathic Medicine,* Baltimore, Maryland: Williams and Wilkins, 1997.

INDEX